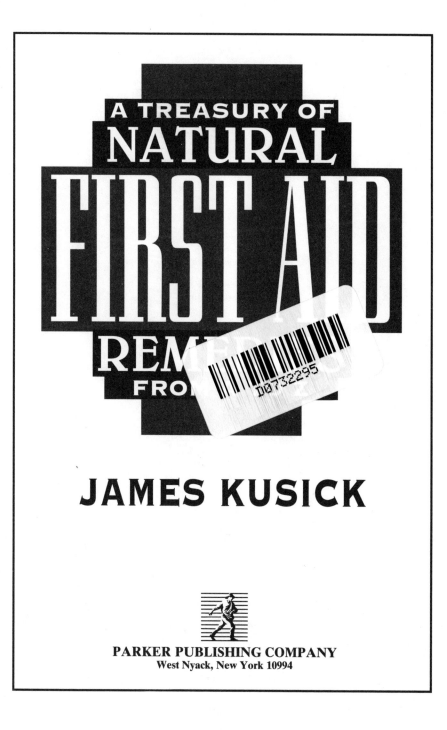

A TREASURY OF NATURAL FIRST AID REMEDIES FROM A TO Z

JAMES KUSICK

PARKER PUBLISHING COMPANY
West Nyack, New York 10994

©1995 *by*
Prentice Hall, Inc.
Englewood Cliffs, NJ

10 9 8 7 6 5 4 3 2 1

Library of Congress Cataloging-in-Publication Data

Kusick, James.
    A treasury of natural first aid remedies from A-Z / James Kusick.
        p.   cm.
    Includes index.
    ISBN 0-13-063173-6.—ISBN 0-13-063181-7 (pbk.)
    1. First aid—Encyclopedias. 2. Naturopathy—Encyclopedias.
RC86.7.K87   1995
615.8'8—dc20   94-30472
                                             CIP

This book is intended as a reference volume only, not as a medical guide
or manual for self-treatment. If you suspect that you have a medical
problem, please seek appropriate medical care.

ISBN 0-13-063173-6
ISBN 0-13-063181-7 (pbk.)

Printed in the United States of America

*This book is dedicated
in loving memory to my mother,
Bessie Opal Kusick.*

ACKNOWLEDGMENTS

As with all major undertakings in life, there are people who give you the support you need to see it through. From my heart I thank my wife, Lovie, for her support, inspiration, dedication, and for taking care of our mundane projects so that I could complete this book. Secondly, a large thank you to Cathryn Anne Rogers for reading through this manuscript several times and for her organizational suggestions. Without either of these two women, this book might still be in my computer.

A very special thank you to my dear friends, Carey Reams, John Christopher, Bernard Jensen, and other mentors whose knowledge inspired me to accomplish my life's task. Their knowledge has helped me bring this book to life and into other people's lives.

In addition, I want to thank the publisher's editor, Douglas Corcoran, for his helpful advice and suggestions.

TABLE OF CONTENTS

A

• 1 •

B

• 17 •

C
• 67 •

D
• 89 •

E

• 97 •

F

• 107 •

G

• 127 •

H
• 133 •

I
• 157 •

L
• 165 •

M

• 169 •

N

• 183 •

P

• 189 •

R
• 197 •

S
• 203 •

T
• 227 •

U

• 241 •

V

• 247 •

W

• 251 •

Y

• 255 •

APPENDICES
• 259 •

INDEX
• 301 •

INTRODUCTION

With the wealth of information currently available regarding "Natural Medicine," much of it conflicting, it is easy for the layman to become confused and give up.

One book may recommend large doses of vitamins while another states that large doses of vitamins are dangerous. There are some herb books available which list the specific herb and then the conditions it will benefit. While this is helpful to someone who is familiar with the different healing herbs, for those not as well-versed the work may simply sit on the shelf and never be used. When one has a crisis, it is far too complicated to search through volumes of herb lore to find what may help.

I was prompted to write this book as a practicing naturopath because many of the emergency calls I've received could have been handled by the callers themselves had there been a clear, simple alternative.

A Treasury of Natural First Aid Remedies from A-Z lists specific complaints alphabetically and then gives several optional remedies, including common kitchen ingredients such as garlic, olive oil, and cayenne which can be used effectively in many instances. For example, if you have an abscess, you would simply look under "A" and find a concise description of the problem and several ways to treat this condition such as apple cider vinegar, witch hazel, or cayenne pepper with the proper dosage given for each.

Another benefit of this book is its cost-effectiveness. In this era of spiraling health care costs, it is wise to be as responsible as possible for your own health. Who can afford to run to the doctor for every small complaint? This work can help you with natural remedies for common problems that, in many cases, cost only a few cents.

A Treasury of Natural First Aid Remedies from A-Z is not written to replace your doctor. Its purpose is to be a handy home-reference guide which can help you cope naturally and quickly with many of life's emergencies.

HOW TO USE THIS BOOK

The best treatment for disease is prevention. Healthy eating, regular exercise, stress management, adequate sleep and rest, a loving, supportive family and social life all contribute to well-being. However, there are times when this can't or doesn't happen. That's why this book was written.

Hopefully, after using the natural remedies suggested in this book for your first aid and acute conditions, you'll become interested in making some lifestyle changes that will help manage or prevent these illnesses from occurring again.

LAYOUT

This book is intended to be a first line of defense against common health problems and first aid situations. This reference guide lists each condition in alphabetical order followed by appropriate natural remedies. Please take a moment to review the major elements for each entry.

First Step: Note the *Description* of the type of injury, infection, or condition under the listing.

Second Step: Note the type of *Action* recommended, such as, how to clean the injury before applying the treatment.

Third Step: Times when the condition can be dangerous, I call attention to it with a 'Warning.' I advise to immediately seek professional medical help.

Fourth Step: Select the *most available remedy* listed under one of the four headings: Kitchen Remedies, Herbal Remedies, Other Natural Treatments, and finally Commercially Prepared Remedies, which include nutrients, herbs, and homeopathic products.

The first remedy listed in each category is the best one to use for that particular health problem. The other listed treatments are also effective if the first one is unavailable or doesn't work for you. I have purposely given you several therapies to choose from in case you don't have or can't find the first few in your local stores.

Rule of thumb: If the particular remedy you have chosen does not help in about 30-40 minutes, then switch to another remedy.

KITCHEN REMEDIES

These are foods, herbs, and spices that can be used if you don't have the specially indicated herbs or commercial products on hand. For example, you can use onions, garlic, and carrots for boils, meat tenderizer for bee stings, and spices like ginger and sage for nausea, food poisoning, and indigestion. Some of the herbal remedies suggested, like peppermint tea, are sometimes common foods found in your cupboard or grocery store.

HERBAL REMEDIES

This category lists the most convenient, easy-to-apply herbal remedies. They are more potent than kitchen herbs or spices and are available in most health food stores. While most of these herbs are used in tea form, they are also available as gels, tinctures, oils, ointments, capsules and tablets. If you are an amateur herbalist, you may be growing some of the herbs I mention in your garden. If so, you can substitute fresh herbs for dried ones. Generally speaking, use three times as much fresh plant as you do the dried.

OTHER NATURAL TREATMENTS

This section lists any miscellaneous, non-commercial treatments that may be useful for your particular ailment or injury. Therapies range from soak baths to helpful vitamins and minerals.

COMMERCIALLY PREPARED HERBAL REMEDIES

To make first aid and self treatment for common health problems easier for you, I have included a list of commercially prepared products I have used with much success over the years. These products include combinations of herbs, vitamins or minerals, or herbs mixed with nutrients. These remedies should be available from your nearby health food store or large food stores.

I have also found combination and single homeopathic remedies to be helpful. Like herbs, homeopathic remedies may not be readily available in most homes. However, they can also be purchased through a health food store or an alternative health care provider.

There are many more natural remedies that work for each problem besides what I have mentioned. But I've limited my suggestions to therapies most people have on hand or can easily purchase at the health food store. I have stayed away from the more exotic and hard to find remedies to make your purchases easier.

CHOOSING THE BEST TREATMENT FOR YOU

The treatments I've suggested work well for most people. However, when choosing a remedy remember that everyone is slightly different in how their bodies respond. I've had some people with abscesses find the drawing effects of freshly sliced potato superior while others responded better to cayenne. If you have a remedy working for you, continue using it. In some cases you may want to apply several suggested remedies at the same time, if available, to the same condition in different areas to see which one works best. For example, you might take an herb by mouth, apply a vegetable poultice, and later do a soak bath.

While most natural treatments are safe, there are times when you shouldn't use them. Pregnancy and nursing are two times when you should avoid any unnecessary medicines—natural or otherwise. If you are ill while pregnant, consult with your physician before taking anything or performing any natural treatments. Children and those already taking medication should also be careful when taking remedies. To make this task easier for you, I have inserted warnings about particular treatments when applicable.

Usually natural treatments such as those outlined in this book will not cause any adverse reactions. However, if at anytime you react to one of the remedies I've suggested, stop taking it immediately. Consult with a practitioner versed in natural medicine for feedback. Also, remember to **avoid** remedies you know you are allergic to. Sometimes people who are severely allergic to a particular substance have serious, sometimes life threatening reactions called anaphylaxis. If this happens, rush the person to the hospital immediately. To minimize this kind of thing from happening, always ask the person you're treating if they're allergic to anything. If they're unconscious, check to see if they're wearing a medical alert bracelet or necklace.

If you are treating someone who is unconscious or having seizures, you should never try to give them any substances by mouth. Instead read the Application Section that follows for suggestions in these cases.

TAKING NATURAL REMEDIES

The following discussion is divided into herbs, commercially prepared remedies, and homeopathic remedies and other natural treatments. In general, instructions on how to take or apply each natural treatment are given for the best results. Follow these directions throughout this book unless otherwise stated.

The dosages for herbs, homeopathic remedies, nutrients, and other natural substances are given for an average adult. If you are excessively over- or underweight, please adjust doses accordingly. As a general rule, children ages 5 to 12 years old should be given half of the adult dosage. Infants and toddlers up to 4 years of age should receive one-quarter the amount taken by an adult. Like adults, if a child is unusually small or large for his age, adjust his dose accordingly. For very small babies who are nursing, often the mother can take the remedy and the child will receive the substance through the breast milk.

You may find that you need to increase the number of times you take a remedy for a few days if the problem is severe. Continue the increased dosage until you begin to feel better and then reduce the dosage amount. You may take any of the liquid or herbal extracts either at room temperature or warm them up slightly.

As you begin to feel better over the next few days, slowly reduce the amount of herbal remedy you have been taking. In the first 1-3 days reduce the remedy by half for liquids or 1 capsule or tablet. If you are still feeling better, then reduce the amounts again by half for another 2-3 days. During this time period, if the symptoms return, go back to taking the amount that made you feel better and take that amount for a little longer period before you begin the next level of reduction.

NATURAL DISINFECTANTS

These substances are usually mentioned under the "Action" section. Disinfectants are used to clean out wounds and prevent most infections before applying the suggested treatment. Many remedies are natural disinfectants themselves. Primary disinfectants are apple cider vinegar, olive oil, witch hazel, cayenne pepper, garlic, lemon, onion, and cloves. Before using a disinfectant and remedy, you can also wash out the wound with a natural soap and water.

If you do not have any of the mentioned disinfectants, you may use cabbage which contains repine, a natural antibiotic, or carrots which pull the poisons out. Juice, finely chop, or dice the secondary disinfectant and apply to area. Keep the poultice on for a few minutes before applying a remedy, or wrap the remedy up with it.

Health food store disinfectants are available in ointments, such as First Aid by Natra-Med or BF&C from Nature's Way. Useful herbal liquid disinfectants are extracts or tinctures of myrrh, taheebo, red raspberry, cayenne, black walnut, or lobelia. Garlic or clove oil, or Dr. Tichenor's are also effective.

HERBS

Tincture, extracts, or liquid drops are the best and easiest form to take and apply to an injured area. This is especially helpful for children, older adults, or anyone where swallowing is a problem. If the remedy tastes "bad," then take it with honey or two to four ounces of natural fruit juice. **WARNING:** Never give honey to children under the age of one year. Honey sometimes contains botulism spores. While this isn't a problem for older children and adults, it can be fatal for babies. Some herbs given on an empty stomach may cause a little nausea; if so, try to give a little food or juice beforehand when possible.

There are many different ways to prepare and administer herbal remedies. Basically there are three different forms of herbs: water based (such as teas), alcohol based (such as tinctures), and fresh or dried herbs. Vinegar can be substituted for alcohol in some tinctures and glycerine is a solvent that's somewhere between alcohol and water. Because water extracts different substances from herbs than alcohols, there are times when a tincture is preferred over a tea and vice versa. A tincture also has a longer shelf life than a prepared tea because of alcohol's preserving qualities. However, there are times when teas or alcohol-free extracts should be used. Avoid giving children, pregnant or nursing women, and alcoholics or recovering alcoholics tinctures.

Throughout the book, I have indicated how and what form of herb to take and when. Below are instructions on how to prepare and/or take each type of herbal remedy.

LIQUIDS If you choose to use an herbal liquid like an oil or tincture, you can take these liquids straight or mask their sometimes disagreeable taste with another substance like fruit juice, or dilute them in cold or hot water. If you take these herbal preparations in hot water like a tea, natural sweetener is optional.

One ounce of tincture equals about the potency of one ounce of the powdered herb. A few drops will be equivalent to 1/2 cup of tea. As a general rule, take 10-20 drops of tincture or extract, or 3-5 drops of oil, 2-3 times daily for normal problems. For more severe problems take this amount every 1-2 hours unless otherwise indicated. Most remedies are listed separately with a few combination suggestions. But you can combine several herbs for stronger effect if so desired.

If giving these remedies to a small child, you may also include any of these remedies in the baby's bottle along with fruit juice to cover the taste. Remember to follow dosage suggestions for children as stated above.

CAPSULES Take 2 capsules 2-3 times daily or more often if your problem is severe or acute, like 2 capsules every 2 to 6 hours. To convert capsules into a tea, open 1-2 capsules into a cup, add hot water, place saucer on the top, and steep about 5 minutes. Remove saucer and either drink the tea down to the sediment or strain it before consuming. If you use 2 capsules or more, the residue can make a second weaker cup of tea by adding more hot water. Then throw this residue out. Natural sweetener is optional.

TEAS There are many different ways to prepare a tea, meaning a hot liquid containing a medicinal herb. Teas are best when trying to extract water-soluble substances from a plant. One type of tea, called a decoction, is made from the hard or woody parts of a plant such as the bark, inner bark, or roots. The extra boiling time needed to make a decoction ensures that you remove all of the soluble, therapeutic compounds in the herb.

To make a decoction you must first boil one or more cups of water. Add two tablespoons of the selected cut-up herb per cup of water. Gently boil in a pot on the stove for 5-10 minutes. Then remove the pan from the heat and let the contents steep for 25-35 minutes. After steeping, strain the tea and save any plant matter to use again for a second batch of weaker tea. Repeat the boiling process with the leftover herbal residue, strain the tea, and discard the herbs. Mix both batches of tea together, adding a little honey to sweeten, if desired, and drink as directed.

You can also make herbal tea like you do regular tea. This tea, called an infusion, is used to prepare the leafy parts of herbs. The essence of the herb is extracted by water **without** boiling. Like making tea, you pour a cup or more of hot water over a teaspoon of a dry herb (powdered, ground, chopped, or leaf) in a mug or teapot, put a lid over the mouth of the container and let the liquid steep for 10-20 minutes covered. Strain off the herb or remove the bag and drink or store. To residues you can add more hot water later for a weaker second cup, then discard the herbs making your next cup from new herbs.

You can drink this infusion as a tea, hot or room temperature. You may add a natural sweetener such as honey, fructose, or fruit juices. If you are using fresh herbs, use one tablespoon of plant to one cup of water.

Sometimes you'll want to make a cold infusion, particularly with plants whose constituents are sensitive to heat. In that case, use cold water, juice, or even milk instead of hot water. (Avoid milk if you are allergic to it or are lactose intolerant.) Use the proportions mentioned above and let the mixture sit in a well-sealed earthen ware container for about eight hours. When you're ready to drink this infusion, treat it as you would a hot infusion: strain and add any sweeteners if you wish.

For either a hot or cold infusion, drink one cup 2-3 times daily or as needed. If the tea is too strong you may dilute it by adding extra hot or cold water. For younger children you can administer the tea in a juice bottle.

If you feel it will be easier for you to make several cups of a tea at once, combine one tablespoon of the selected dried herb (three times this amount if using fresh herbs) with about 2-4 cups of water in a sauce pan and heat with a lid on. Then turn off the heat, keep covered, and steep for 10 to 20 minutes. Strain, discarding residue. Infusions don't have a very long shelf life. You can place the extra tea in an air-tight container and store in the refrigerator for about 3-5 days. If the tea looks, smells, or tastes bad or gets moldy, toss it out.

POULTICE   Bulk herbs or the spices, vegetables, and fruits in your kitchen can be applied directly to injured or diseased body parts as well. One way to do this is as a poultice. Chop, grate, or slice the recommended vegetable or herb. Then make a paste by mixing it with warm water, vegetable oil, olive oil, or wheat germ oil and apply to the affected area. Also, capsules can be opened or tablets crushed and mixed into a paste.

The poultice is applied directly to the injured area or placed inside a natural cloth like cotton, wool, flannel, or linen and placed on the body. Tri-fold the cloth with the opening to the outside so that the bandage can be opened easily and fresh poultice can be applied without disturbing the wound or changing the bandage. The poultice can be held in place with a longer piece of cloth and tied, pinned, or taped to hold the poultice pack in place. You can also secure this mixture with a bandage or gauze and tape.

Change the poultice every 1-4 hours until the symptoms improve and then about every 4-6 hours or overnight as needed. If symptoms are severe, you can apply the poultice as often as every 1/2 hour until acute symptoms subside. Then follow the above directions. Continue using the poultice three times per day for several days after recovery to provide your system additional healing support. You can also mix any extra chopped, grated, or sliced herbs or vegetables you use in your poultice in with other foods, soups, or juices for internal help several times daily.

FOMENTATION   Strictly speaking, a fomentation is an extremely hot, moist compress placed on the body. In fact, normally they are so hot that a bath towel must separate the skin from the fomentation.

When I refer to fomentations, I'm talking about the essence of the herb, usually in liquid or oil form, applied by cloth or directly to the affected area. An example would be warm apple cider vinegar or liquid mullein soaked into a cotton towel. Other times, after you have drunk a tea or extract, you can add any leftovers to a cotton cloth and apply it to the area. This makes the herb work double time.

These fomentations are very easy to prepare. After soaking the towel or cloth, squeeze it to remove the excess liquid and apply to the chest, leg, or other injury or diseased part. Keep the towel or cloth moist by adding the liquid herb to the cloth, or redampen the cloth by immersion and reapply. If removing the cloth will open the wound, just moisten the cloth and leave it on until it comes loose without tearing the area.

The suggested herbs can also be prepared and added to an enema or vaginal douche bag and retained (implanted) in the area. See "Other Natural Treatments" for descriptions and instructions.

COMMERCIALLY PREPARED HERBAL REMEDIES

DOSAGE INFORMATION: The commercial combination herbal and homeopathic remedies listed in the book have been prepared for your ease and convenience. These products allow you to take complex mixtures of herbs, nutrients, and other natural substances in effective quantities so you don't need to figure it out yourself. The amount to be taken is listed directly on the container as recommended by the manufacturer. In some instances, however, I have made additional suggestions for specific conditions.

OTHER NATURAL TREATMENTS

Besides my mainstay remedies found in the kitchen and herbs, there are a variety of other natural treatments you can use. They range from vitamins and minerals to simple treatments you can do at home. Below are descriptions of more complex therapies suggested such as douching, enemas, fasting, implants (vaginal and rectal), slant boards, and soak baths. Sometimes these treatments incorporate herbal products into them, other times they do not. Throughout the book I will tell you when you need to use special ingredients or herbs. But the basic instructions on how to do each treatment are listed below.

DOUCHE   This is a warm solution of water with liquid herbs like the juice of 1/2 lemon, 50 percent diluted apple cider vinegar, liquid trace mineral, or a tea of yellow dock that gently washes the vaginal area as a cleansing and healing bath. This method is used to cleanse and purify the area from infections and old residues. This should not be done routinely, but reserved for special instances. The one exception to this rule is the holding vaginal implant; this is great to do a few times a month for strengthening the vaginal area with healing herbs. You can even leave the implant in overnight and rinse it out in the morning.

Visit your local drugstore to purchase a douche bag or bulb.

ENEMA   An enema is a simple and effective home remedy that helps to quickly release poisons and pressure in the colon so you can feel better. All you need is an enema bag and hose (available at most drugstores), water, and some privacy. Enemas can be used in emergencies when sick with cold, flu, fever, colic, gas, nausea, dysentery, or headaches, and to help cleanse the body of toxins that may interfere with the healing process. Enemas are best used at the first sign of illness to prevent further complications.

Try to use distilled or spring water to avoid exposing your colon to potentially contaminated tap water. Depending on where you live, your tap water may contain chlorine, fluoride, or even pesticides. **Warm water** is best for **quick release** of the toxic waste matter. But **cool water** is best when you want **to hold** the herbal enema (implant) or other suggested enema mixture for a time to loosen the harder fecal matter and heal the area better.

To begin, fill your enema bag with the ingredients for your particular ailment. If nothing special is mentioned, then use water. Make sure the valve on the enema hose is closed so the water in the bag won't leak out. Hang the enema bag about two feet above your body. You may lubricate the nozzle with natural vegetable oil for easy insertion. Never force anything up your anus as the inner surface of the anal and rectal regions is very delicate and easily injured. If you're having troubles inserting the enema nozzle, stop, try to relax with deep breathing, and attempt to do it again.

Place something soft on the floor, if there is a hard surface, to take the strain off your knees and a towel on that to catch accidents. Then kneel down with your head lowered, insert nozzle gently into your anus, lean forward on your elbows with your head still down and let the water in **slowly.** If cramps occur, stop the flow by compressing the control valve, take a few deep breaths and begin again when the cramp ceases. The important thing is not the volume of water but the holding time.

Continue doing this until you feel the pressure is becoming uncomfortable, then expel. Repeat procedure until the bag is empty. You do not have to take the whole bag at one time. You only want enough water released into the colon to give you an urging similar to a bowel movement. This may only require a small amount of water depending on your system and needs. You may want to vary your position while giving yourself an enema. Try lying for five minutes on each side: left, back, right, then back and left side. This may not be possible at first due to the urging to evacuate, but it will become easier to do with time and practice. You may use a slant board to help retain the liquid (see "Slant Board" below).

When you first begin using enemas, you may only hold a small amount of water in your rectum at a time. This is due to the hardened, compressed fecal matter in the rectal area. As you dislodge, loosen, or uncork the fecal matter in the rectum you create room so more matter can move down. You'll be able to hold more water later. Sometimes you may retain the water for awhile. Do not be alarmed; the colon also needs fluid. One reason we have poor bowel movements is from not drinking enough water. One of the colon's jobs is to reabsorb fluids and nutrients. You may release later. You can also use herbs from the "Constipation" section to help clear and heal the upper tract. Later you can use the herbal implants to give additional help. See the section on rectal implants below.

For chronic or long-term ailments, administer an enema two to three times during the first and second weeks to remove the heavier toxins. During the following third and fourth weeks, use an enema 1-2 times and then as needed. By using enemas only as you need them, you will prevent them from becoming habit forming. If you have problems with constipation, see other suggestions under the "Constipation" section.

A special type of enema, called a releasing enema, is used to simply flush the heavy toxins from the system as quickly as possible. Therefore you do not use herbal remedies here. Instead use plain warm distilled or spring water. You may add a teaspoon of baking soda or the juice of 1/2 of a fresh lemon **only,** (strain seeds) no artificial lemon. This will aid the urging action and purify the area. Then proceed as stated above.

FASTING   It is best, sometimes, not to keep loading your body with food when you're sick as it may compound the problem. The main purpose of fasting is to help clean the body of years of accumulated toxic wastes and to let the body rest. In these cases, I recommend you try a short fast. Since most people have hectic schedules, it is best **not** to fast with just water. Instead use water along with fruit and vegetable juices, but no solid foods. Pick a time when you can slow down enough for resting. Do this recommended fast 1-2 times a month.

Begin with a 1-3 day water, fruit, and vegetable juice fast. If you plan to fast longer, visit with a professional trained in therapeutic fasting. Drink 4 ounces distilled water every hour on the hour. A minimum of 12 ounces of a variety of juices should be taken daily. Alternate 4 ounces of fruit and vegetable juice when you desire them. Juice is to be drunk on the half hour (example: 8:30 and 10:30) of the time you want them, but the water is each hour (example: 8:00, 9:00, 10:00, etc.) for 10 hours. The juices will keep your nutrients and electrolytes up and the water will flush out the toxins.

How you break a fast is as important as how you do the fast itself. Do not try to eat normally after fasting for a few days; this will reverse all the therapeutic effects of the fast. Break the fast slowly by eating solid watery foods the first day, such as apples, oranges, fresh homemade soup, an avocado, or a baked potato. Gradually add more solid food like poached eggs or soft, hot grain cereals on the second day. Then work your way to your normal diet, taking as many days to break as you fasted.

IIMPLANTS

Preparation
Implants are usually herbal preparations that are inserted into an orifice in the body such as the rectum or vagina. To make an

implant, use about 1/2-1 teaspoon of tincture, extract, or other liquid concentrate. Milder herbs like aloe vera can be used directly or diluted a little. The stronger herbs may cause irritation and the urge to expel. If using capsules, open them and pour into a cup, add hot water, steep with the saucer on top for a few minutes, strain, and add to the implant water.

You can also steep 1/2 cup of strong bulk tea in about 2 cups of water for about 5 minutes. Strain and add to about 2-3 cups of cool distilled or spring water. Add less water if the implant is hard to retain.

Rectal Implant

A rectal implant is like a mini-enema, except that you want to *retain* a small amount of the herbal solution for a longer period of time so the herbs will have a greater healing effect in the rectum. It may be helpful to perform a releasing enema with half a bag of warm water first to flush out any lower bowel matter before doing the implant. This also eases the bowel pressure urges to expel the implant.

The rectal implant is done much like an enema (see above). At first there may be urges to expel too soon, but if you use small amounts of herbs, in about 2-4 cups of water and do deep breathing, no pushing, you should be all right.

Vaginal Implant

This method can be used in the vagina for various ailments. To do an implant take in a total of 1 pint of the herbal tea in your vagina, holding in as much as you can until the pint is used up. Lay on each side, on your back, or lay in a slant position on a slant board (see "Slant Board" below) or with a pillow under your hips. You can sleep or read for the amount of time you want to retain the solution, then expel or keep in overnight. In the morning use a vinegar douche to clean out the vagina. This can be done a few times a week during an infection to heal and strengthen.

This implant or the vinegar rinse is also good after intercourse. You can use the herbs suggested in the "Vaginitis" entry. By using vaginal implants, you are gaining herbal support and healing both internally and directly on the problem area.

SLANT BOARD   When taking an enema or implant you can also lay in a slanted position with your head down on a slant board. You can make a slant board by placing one end of an ironing board on a chair rung and the other end on the floor. Adjust height for comfort up to 18 inches high. Lay down with your head at the lower end of the board after administering the implant. Try to remain still for 10-20 minutes if possible. You can sleep, read, or visualize yourself getting well during this time. Later expel the solution. This can be done a few times a week to heal and strengthen the lower half of the colon.

SOAK BATH   A soak bath is a great relaxing tonic for the whole body. The heat opens the pores in the skin and encourages elimination of bodily toxins through the skin and into the water. Soaking is also great for various skin problems, hemorrhoids, varicose veins, genital problems, and relaxing the entire body for sleep. It's great for preventing prostate problems as well.

You can add appropriate herbs, one or more, to your soak bath for these various problems as suggested under each condition in the book. Tinctures or teas work well. You can also add steeped herbs in your bath by placing some bulk herbs in a clean sock tied at the end. Place the sock under the running bath water and use it during the bath as a wash cloth. One cup of epsom salt, aloe vera, apple cider vinegar, or baking soda are also added to baths depending on the trouble.

If not used to hot baths, begin slowly by soaking for 5 to 10 minutes at a time and work your way up to a maximum of 20 minutes. Fill the tub with comfortably hot water suited to your body (not above 106°F). If the water is too hot it may draw blood from the brain and cause weakness and dizziness.

Sipping warm tea with a little honey or fruit juice added will keep your energy and keep blood sugar up. When you finish soaking, sit on the side of the bathtub or stand up slowly so you won't get dizzy. Follow your hot bath with a cool bath or shower for a few minutes to close your skin's pores. Dry off, dress warmly, and if possible rest afterwards as it will revive and refresh you. Better yet, have your bath right before bedtime to help you sleep. **WARNING:** This treatment is not recommended if you are very young, very old, weak, anemic, have a tendency to hemorrhage, or have a severe organic disease.

APPENDIX SECTION

Located at the back of this book are several charts, a *Quick Reference Chart* that lists all the health problems covered and offers a limited list of remedies, a *Herbal Helper Chart* that lists the most commonly used herbal remedies and what problems they aid, an Herbal Shopping List that offers the most useful herbal remedies for a variety of problems, and a Glossary.

The Herbal Shopping List is provided so you may make a photo copy, check off the herbs you need, and take it to the health food store for easy purchasing. This saves you and the health store clerk the time, embarrassment, and hassle of trying to pronounce or read your handwriting.

HELPFUL SOURCES AND RESOURCES

If the health store does not carry herbal remedies, then ask them to please carry them. As more people use this book, or others like this one, and ask for such remedies, the more they will have it in stock. Like any business, they operate on the old law of supply and demand.

For more professional help for chronic problems see your doctor or a natural health care practitioner. If you don't know of any professionals trained in natural medicine, begin by checking with friends and your local health food stores. You can also look in the Yellow Pages under Naturopath, Homeopath, Herbalist, Holistic Practitioner, Nutritionist, or Osteopath for help. Also remember that more allopathic medical doctors are using these natural approaches in their practice so make some inquiries.

There are many different types of natural health caregivers. Education, experience, and expertise can vary greatly among these practitioners. It's up to you, the consumer, to ask intelligent questions about their knowledge and experience. If you're not sure where to turn, see the referral list in the appendix. Here I give phone numbers and addresses of professional organizations specializing in various aspects of natural medicine. They will be able to give you the names of doctors and other practitioners in your area.

With so many different types of natural physicians and providers available, it's easy to get confused. Here are some brief descriptions of what some of them do.

Allopathic Physician (MD): Although we are used to referring only to MDs as doctors, in reality there are many different types of physicians. Because of this, the term "allopathic" physician, meaning "other," has been reserved for MDs. As mentioned above, many allopathic physicians are joining the ranks of natural health care providers. Although not initially trained in natural medicine, the "holistic" MD provides the advantage of someone who's familiar with both natural and conventional medicine.

Ayurvedic Doctor: Ayurvedic medicine is a 5000-year-old healing tradition from India that uses diet, exercise, herbs, and other methods. While Western medicine is now predominantly practiced in India, more and more physicians are utilizing the healing principles of Ayurveda in both India and the United States. In some cases, MDs, NDs, and DCs have incorporated Ayurvedic medicine into their practices.

Chiropractor (DC): Originally, chiropractic doctors specialized in disorders of the muscles and skeleton primarily through spinal manipulation. Nowadays, many chiropractors use a variety of therapies to treat musculo-skeletal problems including nutrition.

Naturopathic Physician (ND): A naturopathic doctor trained much like an MD except instead of using drugs or major surgery, his emphasis is on natural treatments such as nutrition, physical therapy, homeopathy, herbs, counseling, natural childbirth, and other therapies.

Oriental Medical Doctor (OMD): An OMD is trained in the therapies and philosophies of oriental medicine. Like Ayurveda, oriental medicine uses many natural therapies but its origins are rooted in China and other Asian countries. Unlike Western medicine, the philosophies, and thus the view of illness, of OM is very different.

Osteopathic Physician (DO): A DO is somewhat like a cross between a MD and a chiropractor. Like MDs, osteopathic doctors can prescribe drugs, perform major surgery, and practice in hospitals. Like chiropractors, a DO's education emphasizes the musculo-skeletal system of the body. Osteopathic techniques usually include gentler manipulations that mobilize the soft tissues of the body, such as muscles. There are, however, many DOs who don't focus on skeletal and muscular problems, but specialize in opthomology (the eyes) or other branch of medicine.

WARNING

Remember there are various serious accidents, heart attacks, or breathing problems that are life threatening and may need more immediate medical emergency help. Immediately call, or have someone call, 911 for an ambulance, para-medic, or a medical emergency unit, or dial the fire department or police for assistance from those who have the background and proper equipment if there is any doubt to the immediate need. Sometimes it may be necessary to transport the injured person to the closest emergency facility. In either case, call or get the nearest help and begin applying the first-aid techniques or remedies you have on hand, including CPR, the Heimlich maneuver, pushing a hot wire off with an object, applying pressure to stop bleeding, or whatever it takes until you can get further help.

Also, I recommend taking the Red Cross emergency CPR training in your area, carry the card on you, and update it as required to stay current to present techniques. We have included the various Red Cross medical emergency techniques right in the alphabetical listing to provide an all encompassing first-aid manual. Please note any additional medical emergency warnings that appear in bold for the most life threatening emergencies. These warnings are to remind you to **call first,** and then to apply recommended first aid.

Even after a serious problem is corrected by on-the-spot first aid help, the person should still be checked by a physician, especially if there has been a severe or chronic, recurring problem, such as heart problems, asthma, blood sugar or insulin problems, epileptic seizure, and so on. Most of these self-help remedies are for short term use until the bleeding stops and heals, or the nausea passes. But the chronic reoccurring problems may need more long-range dietary lifestyle changes and additional natural rebuilding remedies. Poor dietary habits allow toxins to build up gradually over the years in your system and may be the underlying cause of your chronic problems from indigestion, to diarrhea. See a doctor or a natural health care practitioner for a follow-up.

For further natural self-help, please refer to other wonderful books on the subject in the Reference section at the end of this natural remedy guide.

HEALING POWERS IN YOUR KITCHEN

Most people do not think of their kitchen cabinets as medicine chests. Yet the herbs, spices and vegetables you use everyday can be great natural remedies. In fact, many of the seasonings and vegetables, like carrots, onions, and potatoes, we regularly use are also respected medicinal herbs.

Over the centuries people have learned to transform raw plants into more potent forms like tinctures, extracts, oils, powders, and ointments. When you purchase an herb, in whatever form, from a healthfood or specialty store, you may recognize its name. However, this book will also familiarize you with its medicinal qualities. In fact, most medication, both over-the-counter and prescription, is either derived from or synthetically reproduced from plants.

As health care costs rise, it is important to know you have alternative treatments available to you. Botanical and other natural remedies are used throughout the world as viable therapies. Chinese medicine and Ayurveda, medicine from India, use herbs to strengthen and heal the body. Many European and even some American allopathic doctors incorporate herbs and homeopathic remedies into their treatment protocols.

During my years of practice as a naturopath, I have recommended patients use what is available in the kitchen when they cannot get prepared herbs. Often these kitchen remedies are sufficient to resolve the health problem or at least provide relief until professional help is available. So the next time you have a first aid emergency, don't forget to look in your kitchen for help.

The following is a summary of some of the more noted spices or herbs and their therapeutic effects.

ALMOND OIL–This oil is one of the richest sources of protein. It's great for chapped hands and conditions where inflammation or swelling is a problem. Kidney stones and gravel, urinary tract problems, and troubles with the bladder and gallbladder also benefit from this nut oil. For most health conditions, put 10-15 drops of almond oil in hot water or juice and drink. Rub on a few drops of almond extract or oil for skin problems.

BASIL–This sweet, pungent herb is great for stomach complaints, especially cramps and vomiting, and nervous disorders. Arthritis and rheumatism, particularly those cases aggravated by cold, rainy weather, also respond to basil. Dissolve 1/3 teaspoon of basil in a cup of hot water, steep, and strain. If you suffer from an upset stomach, add 1/3 of a teaspoon of sage to the basil tea. (**Caution:** Avoid sage if you are pregnant or nursing.) Sip this tea slowly taking 1 cup 2-4 times daily or as needed.

Basil is also good for tension headaches. For a headache compress, add 1 teaspoon of basil to a cup of hot water, steep a few minutes, and strain. After the tea cools, add 2 tablespoons of chilled witch hazel extract. Apply solution as a compress to the forehead every few minutes or as needed.

CAYENNE–Not only does cayenne stop bleeding instantly, but it fights infections. It helps heal cuts, bites, boils, sores, and even ulcers and internal bleeding. Make a paste by mixing cayenne powder with a little vegetable oil or water and apply it to the injured area. Add some cayenne to a glass of warm water to use as a gargle for sore throats, or relieve mouth sores by holding some solution in your mouth for a few minutes.

Packing cayenne paste around a sore tooth is an excellent way to temporarily relieve a toothache. My wife once had a toothache so painful it woke her up in the middle of the night. After packing the area with cayenne, she went back to sleep in about 10 minutes. Some druggists still sell a dental poultice called Poloris made of red pepper, sassafras, and hops. **Caution:** Cayenne may burn or cause irritation on mucus membranes; e.g., in the mouth, or if applied to a severe infection.

CELERY–Celery's many actions, as a diuretic, sedative, anti-rheumatic, and carminative (relieves flatulence), make it useful for a variety of ailments. Kidney or bladder stones or gravel, gas in the stomach and bowels, rheumatism, neuralgic pains, an upset stomach, nervous headache, and insomnia all respond to celery.

If you have fresh celery, which is best, grate or chop it up and steep in a cup of hot water. Otherwise mix 1/4 teaspoon of celery powder in a cup of hot water. Sip the tea slowly, drinking 2-4 cups a day. For insomnia, you can add 1/2 teaspoon of catnip to your celery tea and drink a cup one hour before bed.

CINNAMON–Cinnamon performs well for nausea, colic, a painful stomach, intestinal gas, diarrhea, chronic indigestion, abdominal discomfort, bloating, heartburn, and vomiting. Mix 1/4 teaspoon of cinnamon powder in a cup of hot water. You may add a little sage or ginger, if you wish. Take 1-2 tablespoons of the tea every so often until you feel relief.

Not only can a cinnamon gargle be used to freshen your breath, but it deodorizes a room too. To give your house a clean, cinnamon-like smell mix 1/4 teaspoon in a quart of warm water. Place the container on a heater during the winter or pour the solution into a spray bottle to mist the room as needed.

CLOVES–This spice is a powerful local antiseptic and anesthetic useful for toothaches. It's also helpful for bronchial disorders, gas, indigestion, and as a breath freshener. To make a tea mix 1/4 teaspoon of clove powder or place 3-5 whole cloves in a cup of hot water. Drink 2-4 cups daily or as needed. To deodorize a sick room, place some clove tea on a hot plate or a few cloves in a vaporizer. For a toothache either pack the tooth with the powder or hold a few cloves against the sore area. You can also drink the tea. Sucking on a clove will help keep your breath fresh. **Caution:** If using clove oil for a toothache, prolonged use may cause serious gum irritation.

FENNEL–Fennel seeds work well for indigestion, intestinal gas, and losing weight. While it's a mild laxative in its own right, fennel can also relieve the gripping effects of harsher laxatives. A few fennel seeds added to your bird's food will tone your bird's intestines. **Caution:** Very large doses can upset the nervous system.

GARLIC–Garlic is one of nature's antibiotics. In addition to its antibacterial effects, garlic also fights viral infections like colds and flu. Garlic stimulates the digestive system, lowers blood pressure when it's high, reduces cholesterol levels, treats respiratory disorders, and is a natural source of sulphur.

The best way to take advantage of garlic's benefits is to eat it on a regular basis. Lemon juice or parsley help cut down on garlic's strong odor. Mix grated or chopped garlic with vegetable oil to apply to lip and mouth conditions like horny swelling (hyperkeratosis), fissures, and ulcers. A garlic poultice eases the discomfort of poison ivy. Make a paste from crushed or freshly juiced garlic, or garlic powder. Then place either concoction between layers of gauze or cotton; keep the poison ivy sores covered for 30-40 minutes.

GINGER–This sweat-inducing spice is great for feverish colds and flu. Additionally, ginger relieves menstrual cramps, minor diarrhea, and colic as well as gas and other intestinal disorders. To take ginger as a tea, mix 1 teaspoon of ground ginger in a pint of water and steep for 10 minutes, stirring occasionally. Take 4 ounces every 1-2 hours or as needed, and less often as you improve.

A ginger poultice, especially when mixed with a little mustard, cinnamon, and warm vegetable oil, helps break up bronchial congestion. Apply this spicy paste to the chest area and cover with a cotton cloth. Leave the poultice on until your chest feels warm and appears pink. **Caution:** Large amounts of ginger shouldn't be used by people with skin problems.

MUSTARD–The stimulating quality of mustard seeds allows this plant to relieve congestion and inflammation as seen in earaches, bronchitis, ulcerated gums, acute sinusitis, and pneumonia. Mustard is also a well-known rubefacient meaning it tends to irritate and redden skin. This explains why it warms you if you have a cold or are chilled due to wet weather.

For a warming foot bath place 1/4-1/2 teaspoon of mustard powder in hot water. While soaking your feet, wrap yourself in a blanket so as not to get a chill. For a chest poultice, steep 1 tablespoon of mustard powder in a cup of warm water and mix with some flour or corn starch to make a paste. You can also make a chest rub by substituting vegetable oil for the flour. To make a tea, dissolve 1/4 teaspoon of mustard powder by itself or with 1/2 teaspoon of sage in a cup of hot water. You can either drink this or moisten a cloth with the tea and apply to the infected area.

ONION–Onion aids sleep, digestion and acid belching, increases urinary output, decreases bronchial congestion by expelling phlegm and mucus, and fights bacterial infections. Either fresh finely chopped onion or onion powder can be used in medicinal preparations. Mix onion with vegetable oil to make a chest poultice for lung congestion. An onion powder paste or poultice can also be used to cool burns and prevent blistering. For a chronic hacking cough, make a cough syrup by mixing 1/4-1/2 teaspoon of onion powder in four ounces of honey or glycerin. Let it stand overnight, if possible, and take 1-2 teaspoons of the mixture several times daily.

PARSLEY–The high iron and manganese content of parsley feeds the blood stream. This bushy green garnish is good for colic and gas pains. Europeans also use it for malaria. Parsley's diuretic actions make it valuable for kidney and bladder problems, and water retention.

For a tea, mix 1 tablespoon of parsley in 1 quart of water and steep for 5 minutes. Take a cupful 3-4 times daily, plain or with a sweetener. For less severe conditions, steep 1/4 teaspoon of the plant in a cup of hot water and drink 1-2 times daily. A parsley poultice can be applied directly over the liver or spleen for conditions involving obstructions. Hot, swollen, inflamed eyes feel better when a parsley tea soaked cloth is placed over them. Eat a handful of parsley to mask the strong odor of onion or garlic. Caution: Don't use medicinal amounts of parsley during pregnancy.

SAGE–This natural and age-old coffee and tea substitute also fortifies health and is superb at preventing disease. Sage is one of the best all-around, simplest on-hand kitchen herbal remedies to use for most health problems. Drinking a spring sage tonic from March 15 to about the last week in May is a great way to clear the body of leftover winter lethargy, especially in cold climates. To make a spring tonic steep 1/2-1 teaspoon of sage in a cup of hot water, then drink 1 cup 1-2 times per day, hot or cold. You may add a little cayenne pepper to warm and stimulate the body. To aid in detoxifying the body, add 1/2 teaspoon of cinnamon to a cup to sage tea.

Medicinally, sage is good for nervous disorders as well as general digestive weaknesses such as indigestion, upset stomachs, gas, colic, and nausea. Sage's anti-infective properties makes it a suitable treatment for salmonella, ptomaine, amoebic dysentery, and feverish colds and flu. One ounce of dried sage simmered in 1 1/2 pints of hot water for five minutes can be used as a general purpose tea or gargle for sore throats and canker sores. Drink 1-2 cups of tea daily for most conditions. If gargling, do so several times throughout the day. To reduce swelling due to sprains or bruises, add a little hot apple cider vinegar to the sage tea and use as a compress. Caution: Do not use sage during pregnancy or if you are nursing.

SALT–Basically salt has been used as a preserver and pickler. However, it is also an excellent emetic (to vomit) when poisons are accidentally swallowed. Dissolve 1/2 tablespoon of salt in a cup of warm water and drink quickly for this purpose. (**Warning:** Do not induce vomiting if someone has ingested a strong acid, strong alkali, or petroleum product. If you are unsure what poison has been swallowed, call the nearest poison control center.)

In addition, salt is great healer for the nose when you have a cold or congestion. Dissolve a few grains of salt in a glass of warm water or mix the salt and water in a dropper bottle. Place several drops of salt solution into your nose, sniffing the salt water solution up into the sinus passages a few times a day. As a gargle for a sore throat, dissolve a little salt in warm water and gargle several times daily. A cloth soaked in salt water wrapped around your neck for 5-10 minutes several times each day also eases a sore throat. Regular table salt may be substituted for Epsom salt to use as a warm fomentation or a soak bath to relieve congestion, draw pus from sores, or soothe sprains and bruises.

A PRIMER ON HERBAL REMEDIES

As I mentioned in the previous chapter, herbs can be found in many places: your kitchen, in the health food store, and even growing wild. That pesky dandelion growing in your lawn is a wonderful liver tonic. Long ago, medicinal herbs provided the backbone of everyday health care. As medicine changed, botanicals were pushed aside in favor of synthetic drugs. This situation is gradually changing again as research reveals the therapeutic value of plants.

We're also discovering the advantage of using whole plants, not just isolated constituents. Many synthetic medications are based on the healing substances found in herbs. When a compound is separated from its source and then magnified, unwanted side effects often occur. Using the whole herb diminishes and even eliminates this problem.

However, herbs should be used with respect and knowledge. Just because herbs are natural, it doesn't mean they are all harmless. Some botanicals in high doses can be poisonous. Others, while safe for most people, may be dangerous to pregnant or nursing women, children, or persons taking certain medications. Notes have been made next to these herbs.

Herbs are wonderful medicines. I encourage you to use them as often as is needed. However, this book is meant to offer short-term solutions. Resist the temptation of taking herbs for long periods of time. Some botanicals lose their effectiveness or may cause unwanted effects if taken for weeks or months on end. If you have an ongoing problem and want to use herbs to treat it, see a professional trained in herbalism.

Finally, not all herbal products you buy are equal. Many different factors affect an herb's potency. Harvest time and place, method of preparation, use of pesticides or not, and how long a plant has been stored all influence effectiveness. For example, an herb that has been cut and dried is much less potent than a tincture or fluid extract. This is why kitchen remedies tend to be weaker than prepared medicinal herbs. Most spices are merely powdered or dried versions of herbs.

Because herbs are more effective the more you know, I've tried to educate you about the remedies you'll be using. Most herbs, because of their complex nature, possess a host of therapeutic effects. So under each condition, I've described why each herb is useful for that particular ailment. See "How to Use This Book" for more details on dosage information.

A PRIMER ON HOMEOPATHIC REMEDIES

Homeopathy is a 200-year-old system of medicine developed by Samuel Hahnemann, a German physician. Like many other natural therapies, homeopathy is enjoying a resurgence as professional associations and educational programs increase. Many people have discovered how useful homeopathy can be for home care too.

Available as little white sugar pills, liquids, ointments, or creams, homeopathic remedies appear to contain not even a trace of substance. Yet the plants, minerals, and animal matter that comprise homeopathic remedies have proven themselves to be powerful medicines.

Unlike conventional medicine, homeopathy helps to realign and stimulate the body's inner healing powers referred to by homeopathic practitioners as the "vital force." Because homeopathy is so different from Western medicine, it's important to understand the laws that guide it.

The first law of homeopathy is "like cures like." This means that a substance which produces particular symptoms when given to a healthy person can be used to treat the same symptoms in a sick individual. For example, *allium cepa* or onion, a plant that normally causes eyes to tear and redden, is ideal for colds where watery, red eyes is a symptom.

Hahnemann decided homeopathic remedies should be administered in very small doses. He did this to avoid the adverse reactions sometimes caused by medications. So homeopathic medicines are diluted to a point where no side effects occur, yet they retain their effectiveness. In fact, the more dilute the remedy, the more powerful it is. Vigorous shaking is another important step in preparing homeopathic remedies. It is believed that this shaking potentizes the remedy as well.

In classical homeopathy, there are two basic ways of prescribing: acute and constitutional. Constitutional homeopathy, a complex and extensive treatment for the body in general, requires the services of a professional trained in homeopathy. For our purposes here, short term illnesses or first aid at home, we will use acute homeopathy.

For the best results, you can't just match a remedy to a disease. To properly self-administer acute homeopathic remedies, you need to closely observe symptoms. For example, every cold is not the same. The quality and amount of nasal discharge, presence or absence of watery eyes, and the patient's general temperament all vary.

You can also use commercially prepared homeopathic remedies. These tablets or ointments are usually a combination of several different homeopathic substances put together to treat a general symptom such as a fever or cough. To make treatment as easy as possible for you, I have suggested several homeopathic products under the "Commercially Prepared Remedies" listed under each condition throughout the book. See "How to Use This Book" for dosage information.

If you want to learn how to administer individual remedies for acute conditions, see the "Reference" section for book suggestions on how to do this. Check with your local health food store to purchase individual homeopathic remedies.

A HEALTHIER YOU

Staying healthy is easier than getting healthier. There are proper rules to follow to keep you well.

Proper attitude is essential. You are a whole person; mind, body, and spirit. Each affects the other. Your mind and spirit must be at peace for the body functions to work in harmony. After working with a middle age lady who had open sores on her right leg for a month to six weeks, her progress was remarkable. Energy levels were up and open sores on her legs were almost healed. I told her that it looked like she could return to work in another week. Two days later I was told that she was too weak to sit up and the sores on her right leg were red, and dark yellow pus was erupting. She had not changed her program. After counseling with her I found an attitude toward her boss to be one of strong resentment. She felt he was looking over her shoulder all the time and putting her down to other workers. She felt she could not say anything because he was her brother-in-law. After talking a while, she realized he had a problem trusting any woman with responsibility. (His mother had left him at the age of three.) With a prayer of forgiveness and offering love to him, she returned home and the healing continued and she indeed returned to work.

Proper clean water drunk in the proper amount at the proper time is the first action for good health. Drinking half of your body weight converted into ounces will keep toxins washed out of your system. Example: A person weighing 150 pounds needs at least 75 ounces of water a day; distilled is best. This is plain water, not teas nor juices, and best to be in small amounts as near hourly as possible. Drinking four ounces at a time will not wash out your blood sugar and electrolytes. If a person weighs under 100 pounds you would decrease the amount to three ounces, and if the body weight is more that 175 pounds you increase the amount to six ounces.

I have found by drinking distilled water a person improves faster. Some say this depletes the body of minerals. I feel if the minerals are lying around unassimilated they are not doing you any good anyway. A person starting on our program usually starts out drinking about forty ounces a day until we see how the pancreas responds.

Break from this routine of water intake half an hour to an hour before and after eating so digestive juices are not weakened. Same reason for the rule of not drinking while eating.

Proper food is essential to fuel our body. Stress and abuse of what we put into them over the years make for different types of problems. No two people carry the same stress load so basic rules may need to be altered from time to time. But the goal is to bring the chemistry into balance. Ideally, eat whole grains and seeds, fresh raw fruits and vegetables with the proper water. Adjustments to the rules are made at times for correction. Think about the different diet programs you have seen throughout the years. Today's diets vary in some degree, but the oldest diet known in the Bible, follows these same principles. I am not here to discuss doctrine, but to say when you follow these principles you may live longer and healthier lives.

Eating is meant to be an enjoyable time. Take time to chew your food at least twenty times a bite. A beloved professor once said make soup with each mouthful. Mealtime is not the time to watch the news nor discipline a child; be uplifting to others and have pleasant and happy conversation at the table. Time to eat and digest your food is important; as a rule I would not eat if I had less than a half hour, or longer, for a complete meal. Look at what this says about our school system.

Microwave ovens are a curse to our bodies. They cook the food from the inside out destroying the enzymes and scrambling energy so the digestive tract does not know what to do with the food. Mothers call complaining about crying, colicky babies. When asked if they are warming the bottle in a microwave, most of the time the answer is yes. If they will stop this the babies usually settle down in days. The waves from the microwave drain our energy even when not in use. This is not a popular theory but after unplugging them and watching the energy levels come up in my clients and family tells me it must be true.

Proper digestion and assimilation are the keys to staying healthy. Putting in the proper foods but not assimilating will not do any good. This is part of the reason for the absence of drinking while eating. You are to chew food till liquid and not wash it down, enlisting digestive enzymes. Chewing gum a few minutes before eating induces the digestive juices to begin flowing. If you have had a heavy meal, chew a stick of gum a few minutes to help digest, but not more than ten minutes. Chewing gum for long periods of time over-works the digestive juices and confuses the stomach which can prevent assimilation.

Proper elimination is very important. Putting the nutrients into the body is vital but just as vital is the elimination. If only one area slips we start on the road of illness. We should have three to five bowel movements a day. The most frequent thing I hear is "I did not have time." The school systems will not allow children time to go to the restroom, plus in a lot cases they would be frightened to go. Leaving processed foods and sweets out of our diet, eating live and wholesome food, and drinking properly will allow elimination to happen automatically. A variety of foods are necessary, and one should eat foods that are in season. The foods are ripe at certain times of the year for a purpose; different kinds of herbs and foods feed different parts of the body. This is one of the purposes of this book. Teenage girls come in with cramps, and when I tell them to eat squash and okra at least three times a week they are horrified. Seeded vegetables feed the reproductive systems of both female and male. Dates, prunes, and okra help the elimination tract, and so much more.

Proper rest, recreation, and exercise are the last three areas I want to touch on at this time. The proper rest and sleep for your body is important for a healthy body. The healthier you are the fewer hours of sleep you will need. Rest and recreation are vital stress management controls. Playtime is important to be able to maintain a productive work load. When possible, be outdoors for the fresh air. Exercise is necessary for keeping proper circulation and elimination throughout the body. Walking is the best type of exercise; remember to breathe in deep and exhale slowly and completely. Remember even God rested on the seventh day.

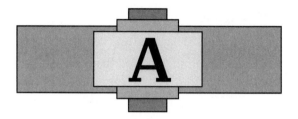

ABSCESS

An abscess, a collection of pus, or decaying material and debris, can be found almost anywhere in the body, such as the lungs, mouth, or even the brain. A wide variety of bacteria, the usual cause of infection, can be cultured from an abscess. Heat, redness, swelling, pain, and sometimes fever are typical symptoms.

Although an abscess may heal on its own, drainage is usually recommended. If this isn't done surgically, the abscess may come to a head, burst and cause the infection to spread. Sometimes headaches occur as the result of an abscess in the mouth or gums. Toxins in the blood, poor food, and indigestion may cause this unpleasant condition.

In this section I will discuss treatments for abscesses found in the mouth or on the skin. If you suspect you have an internal abscess, see your doctor.

ACTION

Wash and clean the infected area with a natural soap and water, then apply a natural disinfectant such as apple cider vinegar, witch hazel, cayenne pepper dissolved in water, lemon juice, salt water, hydrogen peroxide, or rubbing alcohol. Leave the disinfectant on the abscess for a few minutes before applying a remedy. Many of the suggested herbal remedies are also disinfectants.

If the abscess is in the mouth, rinse out the mouth several times daily with a natural disinfectant before applying one of the suggested remedies.

KITCHEN REMEDIES

Aloe Vera–If you're using a live aloe plant, slice open a leaf and place or rub the gel-like innards directly on the abscess several times a day. This works particularly well for small abscesses on the skin. You may want to band-aid a small piece of an open leaf to the infected area. Leave it in place for 12 hours or so. Replace the aloe and bandaid after a shower or as needed. An abscess inside your mouth can be treated with liquid aloe. You can purchase aloe vera concentrate (gel or clear) from a health food store or make your own. Prepare homemade aloe liquid by mixing one to two cups of water and a large piece of aloe plant in a blender at medium speed a few seconds. Fill your mouth with the aloe mixture (homemade or purchased), hold it on the sore area for about five minutes and then spit the liquid out. You can also moisten a piece of cotton batting with this aloe liquid and tuck the cotton up against your mouth abscess. Pour any leftover aloe juice into a small container with a tight lid and refrigerate it until needed again.

In addition, if you have an internal abscess, you can drink aloe as well. Mixed with a little fruit or fruit juice in your blender, aloe makes a refreshing beverage. Drink about 4-6 ounces several times daily.

Cayenne–This natural antiseptic acts as a blood purifier and eases pain. For sores inside your mouth, mix 1/4 teaspoon of cayenne in 4 ounces of warm water, then hold the mixture in your mouth for a few minutes until the pain stops.

You can also use a cayenne paste, made by adding a little warm water or olive oil to a tablespoon of cayenne, for abscesses on the skin. First cover the affected area with a damp cotton cloth, then apply the paste. If too strong or if you are sensitive, the cayenne may burn and cause blisters. If you feel discomfort, quickly wash the cayenne off. Generally speaking, however, clients have reported good results with this remedy, especially those with toothaches.

Wheat Germ Oil, Vitamin E or A–These oils, available in liquid or capsule form, promote healing and soothe pain. Spread any one of these oils on the abscessed area or mouth sore with a disinfected finger or cotton swab. Use 2-3 times a day or as needed.

Cloves–Place a few whole cloves or warm clove tea in your mouth against the abscess for several minutes.

Garlic–Like cayenne, fresh garlic can irritate raw areas on the skin. However, garlic is a superb, natural antibiotic. To prevent discomfort, rub a protective coating of vegetable oil over the infected tissue before applying grated or chopped garlic to the abscess. You can substitute garlic oil for fresh garlic if you like. Add a few drops of this oil to juice and drink throughout the day. Use fresh garlic generously in cooking.

Carrot, Onion, Potato, or Tomato–Grate, chop, or juice any of these vegetables and apply as a poultice to the area.

Raisins–Eat a large handful of raisins 2-3 times daily. Raisins cleanse the blood and are high in iron. You can also mash the raisins and apply them as a poultice to the infected area of the skin.

Thyme or Sage–Most people use thyme and sage as spices. However, both of these herbs are antiseptics helpful in treating infected wounds such as abscesses. Sage also has astringent and anti-inflammatory properties. When combined together in a tea, I have found these herbs especially good for problems with the teeth. **WARNING:** Avoid sage during pregnancy.

Castor or Olive Oil–Rubbing one or both of these oils on your abscess may enhance healing.

SINGLE HERBAL REMEDIES

Chamomile–This herb is not only an antispasmodic and gentle sedative, but also soothes inflammation, eases pain, and promotes wound healing. Take as a tea 2-3 times a day.

Clove or Peppermint Oil–The volatile oils in these plants soothe and heal sores. Apply 3-5 drops of either oil to a piece of cotton and rub the affected area. Use twice a day or as needed.

Echinacea– Echinacea is an antiseptic effective against both bacterial and viral infections almost anywhere in the body. Together with its immune stimulating and wound healing properties, this plant is an ideal natural medicine for abscesses. Take as a tea, 2-3 times a day.

Goldenseal–This is a good infection fighting and immune boosting herb. Take as a tea or in juice 2-3 times a day. **WARNING:** Avoid goldenseal if you're pregnant as it stimulates uterine muscles. Avoid the single herb if you have hypoglycemia.

Myrrh–Myrrh is specific for infections in the mouth and tooth problems. While battling infection and stimulating white blood cells, a vital component of the immune system, myrrh relieves pain. Take as a tea or in juice 2-3 times a day. If you have powdered myrrh, you can moisten it with a little water and pack the infected area.

Black Walnut Extract–This herb helps draw infected matter out of an abscess, as well as heal it. Take as a tea or in juice 2-3 times a day.

OTHER NATURAL TREATMENTS

Soak Bath–If there are a lot of abscesses all over your body or on your arms and feet, then you may want to soak the infected areas in a bath. A hot bath relaxes you, induces sweating (thereby promoting detoxification), and stimulates the immune system. All these actions will help your abscesses heal. Add 1-2 cups of Epsom salts to comfortably hot water.

COMMERCIALLY PREPARED HERBAL REMEDIES

Herbs: Kalmin (antispasmodic); Cal-Silica (natural calcium); BF&C capsules or ointment (rebuilds bone, flesh and cartilage); Pau d'Arco Bark (Fights infections) (Nature's Way); Bone All; Vege-Cal (natural calcium) (Schiff) or Calcium Citrate (Twin Lab). Liquid trace mineral is first aid in a bottle because it is a great all-purpose agent for cleansing and healing.

Homeopathic: Headache & Pain; Injuries; Detoxification; Teeth and Gums (Natra-Bio); Injury & Backache (Medicine from Nature).

ALLERGIES

We typically think of allergies as causing swollen and painful sinuses, headaches, watery eyes, or runny noses. These symptoms are usually the result of pollens in the air resulting in a condition we often call hay fever or rose fever. The truth is an allergy is a heightened sensitivity to almost anything: foods, dust, or molds in your home or office, animal hair, cigarette smoke, and even everyday substances like perfume or paint. An allergic person may react in a number of ways aside from sneezing. Symptoms range from fatigue, rashes, and joint pains to mental haziness and other unexplainable signs.

WARNING: Food allergies sometimes mimic food poisoning. If there is any doubt call your doctor. (See "Food poisoning").

ACTION

If your eyes and sinuses are irritated due to hay fever or other airborne allergens, avoid rubbing your face as much as possible. Decreasing your exposure to things you are allergic to will also help. If you already know what you're probably allergic to, then try avoiding these substances. You can also visit with a professional who administers allergy tests.

Food allergies are more common than we think. If you are aware of any food sensitivities, change your diet by eliminating these items. The most common allergenic foods include wheat, dairy, soy, eggs, tomatoes, citrus fruits, peanuts, and chocolate. Take notice of additives in your toiletry products such as toothpaste, soaps, scented and colored tissue, or toilet paper. Carbon monoxide and other poisonous gases from a heater, furnace, or stove can also cause problems. Mold in humidifiers, old furnaces, window air conditioners, and cosmetics may cause reactions too.

If you suspect you have gastrointestinal candida (a yeast infection in the gut), please see your doctor for a test. Candida may exacerbate allergic reactions (See "Yeast Infections" and "Sinuses").

The following remedies are used primarily for respiratory symptoms.

KITCHEN REMEDIES

Brewer's Yeast–This supplement is great for allergies because of its B vitamins. It is usually available in powder form. Take 1/4 to 1/2 teaspoon in juice, or sprinkled on food or cereal. Because of its taste, for children, add the yeast food or drink in very small amounts and gradually increase to the children's dosage over the next few weeks. **WARNING:** Don't take brewer's yeast if you have a yeast infection or are allergic to yeast.

Horseradish–This old folk remedy is a great cleanser and stimulant. Mix freshly grated or commercially prepared horseradish root with a little apple cider vinegar. This can then be stored for future use.

Begin treatment with 1/3 teaspoon of this remedy 3-4 times daily taken either straight or added to your food. Gradually increase this amount to tolerance. If suffering from a congested chest or cough, you can use the horseradish in a poultice. First spread olive oil on your chest, then apply the grated horseradish and cover with a cotton cloth. A bowl full of horseradish on a table by your bed will ease breathing while you sleep.

Onions–From the same family as garlic, onions possess anti-asthmatic properties. Place these sliced or chopped vegetables in a bowl by your bed. Breathing the fumes will help open up and purify the sinuses.

Salt Water–Called nasal douching in Ayurvedic medicine, inhaling salt water is thought to disinfect the nose and cleanse it of mucus. Put a teaspoon of salt in a pint of warm water and shake well. Sniff up the salt water or use a dropper to put a few drops in your nose if nasal congestion is a problem. If the mixture burns, then dilute the salt water. Also gargle with the salt water several times daily.

Thyme–The expectorant quality of thyme tea helps thin and move mucus out of your lungs and sinuses. It's great when mixed with fenugreek.

Honeycomb–Chew a piece of honeycomb several times daily. If available, it is best to use combs from local bees as this aids your body in assimilating local pollens.

SINGLE HERBAL REMEDIES

Bayberry–Bayberry, an astringent and aid for all mucus membranes problems, helps dry up stuffed noses. Prepare a bayberry solution by emptying one capsule of dried bayberry in a cup of hot water and steep for two minutes. Strain the liquid and allow it to cool. Inhale or place a few drops of this solution in your nose as needed. If your throat or chest are affected, apply a warm compress soaked in bayberry fluid around your neck and chest several times a day.

Eucalyptus Oil–To open up nasal passages, place 3-5 drops of eucalyptus oil in either a pan or a sink of hot water. Then with a towel draped over your head and the container, lean over and breath deeply for 10 minutes. Repeat as needed. You can also add this oil to a humidifier or vaporizer for a long-term effect.

Fenugreek–This herb helps break up and move respiratory mucus. Take as a tea or in juice 2-3 times a day.

Garlic Oil–Garlic's expectorant qualities are useful for mucus build up due to allergies. Put 3-5 drops of garlic oil in juice or food daily. You can also rub some garlic oil on the front of your neck and sinus areas and then wrap the area with a cloth. As always, put vegetable oil on first to avoid irritation.

Lungwort–This is an expectorant which breaks up mucus and offers respiratory help. Make a tea by putting 10-20 drops of the liquid in a juice or open 1-2 capsules in a cup of hot water. Drink.

Marshmallow–This lubricates lungs and mucus membranes and is great for inflammation caused by allergies. Take as a tea or use in juice 2-3 times a day.

Mullein–If you have hay fever, this remedy works very well. Take as a tea, 2-3 times a day.

Myrrh–The expectorant, astringent, and anticatarrhal properties of this plant make it great for hay fever. By stimulating the body's natural defenses, myrrh helps your body cope better with allergies. Take as a tea.

COMMERCIALLY PREPARED HERBAL REMEDIES

Herbs: HAS (Contains ephedra, a natural antihistamine and decongestant. If you are sensitive to ephedra use HAS Fast Acting Formula *without* ephedra.); Breathe Aid; Kalmin (anti-spasmodic); Allergy Care (ephedra); BronCare (epherdrin); Sinustop (pseudoephedrine); or, Red Clover Combination (Nature's Way).

> **WARNING:** Ephedra is a stimulant. Do not take this herb, any derivative of it (epherdrine, pseudoephedrine) or a product containing such directly before bed. Side effects can include insomnia, increased blood pressure, increased heart rate, and anxiety. Do not take this if you are pregnant, have heart disease, hypertension, diabetes, thyroid disease, or difficulty urinating due to an enlarged prostate. Avoid this product if you're taking medication for depressant or blood pressure.

Homeopathic: Allergy; Hayfever, Sinus; Raw Lung; (Natra-Bio) or, Allergy or Sinusitis (Medicine from Nature).

ANXIETY, NERVOUSNESS, OR PHOBIAS

We have all felt fear and anxiety. Most times these sensations are normal reactions to stressful or sometimes dangerous events in our lives. Symptoms may include chest pain or pressure, trembling or shakiness, fear of losing control, a pounding heart, a choking sensation, shortness of breath, dizziness or nausea, increased activity, and lack of concentration.

For some, these feelings are long term and/or so intense they interfere with everyday life. Fears become phobias such as fear of heights, crowds, open spaces, or snakes. Anxiety manifests itself as either debilitating panic attacks or the milder, chronic anxiety disorder.

ACTION

If fears, anxiety, or panic rule your life, seek professional help. If you are occasionally bothered by nervousness and want help to get through those trying times, the following suggestions may help.

First of all, reassure yourself by repeating, "I'm okay, you're okay, everyone is okay. Everything is all right." At the same time try to relax your body by taking deep breaths and letting them out slowly. Sometimes anxiety is caused or exacerbated by a drop in blood sugar or an emotionally upsetting situation like being late for a meeting, getting a traffic ticket, or missing a flight connection.

If you are prone to low blood sugar due to lack of food, carry some hard candy or a little box of raisins with you to keep your blood sugar up until you can eat. If you are very anxious about a meeting or presentation, you may be suffering from a symptom like stage fright or performance anxiety. Determine the cause of your fears. If there are real reasons for your nervousness, take steps to relieve this problem. If the reasons are imaginary, then try to talk it out with a close friend, or professional counselor or minister. Most people worry about things that will never happen or over which they have no control over.

KITCHEN REMEDIES

Candy–To help keep your blood sugar from dropping, carry some hard, suckable candy in your pocket, purse, briefcase, or glove compartment of your automobile. Use naturally made candy.

Fruit–Eat fresh apples, bananas, or grapes. Pre-sliced or dehydrated and bagged fruits are easier when you are on the go. Fruits help keep your blood sugar up.

Fruit Juices–You may make your own fresh juices from blending or using a juicer from apples, bananas, or grapes and then put them in a container with a screw-top lid for easy transporting to the office or use in your automobile. Health food stores also have bottled natural juices.

Raisins–Eating a handful in mid-afternoon keeps your blood sugar from dropping between meals. Store a box in your glove compartment, desk drawer, or in a pocket.

Licorice–This is good for balancing the pancreas and the blood sugar. It is best to get the naturally made licorice from your local health food store. Either purchase licorice that is in small bite sizes or cut up the large strands so that you may suck on it.

WARNING: Don't take licorice if you have a history of high blood pressure or kidney failure. Don't use licorice if you use heart medication called cardiac glycosides (check with your doctor.) Don't take licorice for prolonged periods of time or excessive amounts of it. If you experience side effects such as water retention and high blood pressure, stop taking this herb.

Celery–Chew 1/2 of a celery stick or drink 4-6 ounces of celery juice 1-3 times daily, especially when it's difficult to relax at bedtime. Celery helps feed and calm the nervous system.

Milk–Drink a warm cup of milk before resting. An amino acid called tryptophan helps calm the body.

Sage–Make sage tea as it is a good relaxant and calms the nerves.

SINGLE HERBAL REMEDIES

Cayenne–By strengthening the nervous system, this tea helps combat anxiety. Take 1-2 capsules 1-2 times a day. Keep some in the car, at work or in a pocket. Or, make a tea by putting 10-20 drops of the liquid in juice or tea, or, open 1-2 capsules in a cup of hot or room temperature water, or in juice. Drink 2-3 times a day.

Chamomile–Great for nerves as it is soothing and acts as a mild sedative, especially for children and babies. Make a flavorful tea.

Hawthorn–A good heart tonic that calms palpitations when taken as a tea. **Warning:** If you're suffering from chronic heart palpitations or any other heart symptoms such as chest pain, see your doctor.

Skullcap–This herb is food for the nerves and it calms the system. Make as a tea.

Spearmint, Catnip, or Peppermint–Any of these herbs are good for nerves and can be used for children. Make a flavorful tea.

Valerian Root–Since this is a strong nervine, an herb that calms nervous excitement, it is best not to use for small children under the age of 4. Use as a tea.

OTHER NATURAL TREATMENTS

Calcium (500 mg) or Calcium-Magnesium (500 mg/250 mg)–Take one tablet or capsule 2 times daily with water. Try to take one dose before bedtime. Either of these remedies feed and calm the nervous system.

Vitamin B Complex–This vitamin aids in calming and feeding the nervous system. Take 1 (50 milligrams) capsule once each day. Take these vitamins early in the day. Be sure they are yeast free if you have a Candida infection.

COMMERCIALLY PREPARED HERBAL REMEDIES

Herbs: PC Formula (Helps balances the pancreas and blood sugar.); Kalmin Extract (An antispasmodic good for all types of panic or emotional attacks. You can take the drops directly or in water or juice. Works in a few minutes.); Adren-Aid (Supports adrenal to keep up energy, control nervousness, and regulate the heart and pancreas.); Ex-Stress liquid (Helps regulate the heart and calms the entire nervous system.); Cal-Silica (Provides natural calcium to support the nerves and calms the system.); Fem-Mend, Or Change-O-Life (Aids menopause and emotional balance.) (Nature's Way); or, Rescue Remedy (For shock, trauma, injuries, and various fearful thoughts.) (Bach).

Homeopathic: Raw Pancreas; Adrenals; Raw Female or Male; Nervousness; Headache; Menopause; Emotional; Candida Yeast; PMS (Natra-Bio); or, Fatigue; Menopause; PMS; Tension; or, Headache (Medicine from Nature). For more specific fears like: fear of heights, death, darkness, being home alone, storms, crowds, public places, open spaces, drowning, fire, bridges, confined to a place, or, loosing self-control, etc., see a homeopath trained in these areas.

APPENDICITIS

Pain in the abdomen can be caused by a variety of conditions, such as an ulcer, gallbladder attack, problems in the vagina or ovaries, an intestinal infection, and appendicitis. Inflammation of the appendix, or appendicitis, should be suspected if the person is between the ages of 15-25. Pain from appendicitis typically begins in the middle of the abdomen and spreads to the lower right side. Here the tenderness and tight feeling are well localized and aggravated by movement, sneezing, coughing, or deep breathing. The individual may also experience nausea, vomiting, and recent constipation. A low grade fever may appear later.

Pain in the left groin area is occasionally a symptom also. This is usually due to toxic or congested bowel pressing on the appendix or cecum area. Poor diet and sluggish bowel movements can contribute to this. If pain and fever become noticeably worse, the appendix may have ruptured.

WARNING: If you suspect you have acute appendicitis, get to a doctor or hospital immediately. A ruptured appendicitis can cause serious internal problems which may lead to death. Do not attempt any home remedies or delay receiving proper medical attention.

ASTHMA

The frequency and severity of asthma symptoms among people vary greatly. Some people experience fairly mild, occasional asthmatic attacks with no other symptoms. Others are bothered by coughing and wheezing, punctuated by frightening attacks. An asthmatic attack can begin quickly or develop slowly as respiratory distress worsens. During an attack labored breathing, wheezing, coughing, a tight chest, nervousness, and congested lungs are apparent. Asthmatic attacks can subside quickly or persist for hours or days.

Asthmatics have bronchial systems that over-react to various stresses such as infection, exercise, upsetting situations, irritants such as gas fumes, cigarette smoke, allergies, or even changes in the temperature or barometric pressure. Why this happens, no one is sure. My theory is that asthma is usually due to emotional stress, such as suppressed anger or fear.

> **WARNING:** If you are unable to control an asthmatic attack with prescribed asthma medication, seek appropriate medical attention immediately.

ACTION

During an attack it may help to loosen your clothing, get plenty of fresh air, and keep calm.

Other times, use relaxing herbs like an antispasmodic tincture such as catnip. Have your physician check for gastrointestinal yeast infection, allergies, or mononucleosis.

KITCHEN REMEDIES

Garlic or Onion–These vegetables help clear the bronchial tubes, and fight any secondary infections that may occur. Garlic eases the bronchial spasms of asthma as well. Add a liberal amount of these aromatic vegetables to your diet, or use garlic oil (available in the health food store) in a tea. Chop or dice the vegetables mixing them with a little olive oil. However, first rub chest and neck with olive or vegetable oil, then apply the mixture. Either warmed vegetable can also be applied to the bottom of feet after spreading a little olive oil first, then cover the feet with clean, white cotton socks. If you don't want to go to that trouble, use garlic oil instead. We were called after midnight about a three month old baby having trouble breathing. The mother did not have any liquid herbs, so I told her to put olive oil on the baby's feet. Then rub a sliced piece of garlic on the baby's feet and if the baby was not any better in thirty minutes take her to the hospital. Noon the next day the mother called and said the baby had relaxed and was sleeping peacefully in twenty minutes after application. To assist in easier breathing place a dish of either or a combination of garlic and onions by the bed at night.

Horseradish–Use either the premade product or freshly grate some horseradish and add in a little apple cider vinegar. Take 1/3 of a teaspoon in a little soft food and hold it for a few minutes in your mouth, then swallow it. Gradually increase the amount you take so that your system can become accustomed to the horseradish. You can also make a poultice to spread over the chest area. Horseradish clears up the bronchial tubes.

Sage and Ginger–Take either as a tea or use as a poultice. Sage soothes the lining of the lungs and ginger helps stimulate blood flow to the respiratory system.

Apple Cider Vinegar–This performs as an antiseptic and fights infection. Take 1 teaspoon of this in 4-6 ounces of water or apple juice. Drink it slowly while resting. Repeat as need.

SINGLE HERBAL REMEDIES

Eucalyptus–Works great as an antibiotic and antiseptic vapor. Put 10-20 drops in hot water, then drape a towel over your head breathing in deeply. Place a few drops in your humidifier to aid easier breathing especially during the night. You can also add other herbal oils such as garlic, mullein, chamomile, or fenugreek to the preparation. Eucalyptus breaks up congestion in the lungs when used as a hot pack. Warm the oil and spread over the chest, then apply heat with hot towels or a heating pad.

Mullein–Great for soothing the mucus membranes of the respiratory system and clearing lung congestion. Mix a few drops of antispasmodic tincture in the tea. You may use the oil as a hot pack by spreading it over the lungs. Then apply heat with hot towels or a heating pad.

Fenugreek–This herb is great for all mucus and lung conditions. You can also use fenugreek as a fomentation. Make a tea every one to two hours for 3 times if needed.

Pleurisy Root–Great for relieving mucus, and the painful breathing caused by spasming bronchials. Make a tea.

Elecampane–Dissolves thick phlegm, mucus, and is especially good for chronic asthma. Make a tea. Foment the chest, if you wish, for additional help.

Peppermint, Skullcap, or Valerian Root–All of these calm the body's system and soothe a tight chest. Add 10-20 drops to 1 cup of water and drink 3-4 times daily. You may foment the chest area with these herbs.

OTHER NATURAL TREATMENTS

Soak Baths–A great relaxing tonic for the whole body. The heat expands the skin and inner body tissue drawing the toxins to the skin's surface and into the water. While filling the tub with hot water add single or combination of herbs mentioned above. Tinctured or liquid teas are very good here. Use 1-2 cups of Epsom salts or 1 cup of aloe vera, apple cider vinegar, or baking soda.

COMMERCIALLY PREPARED HERBAL REMEDIES

Herbs: HAS (breathing help); Comfrey-Mullein-Garlic Syrup; Breath-Aid; Kalmin (antispasmodic); Fenu-Thyme (releases mucus and congestion); Ex-Stress (for nerves); Nature's Way; or, Rescue Remedy (for shock and anger) (Bach).

Homeopathic: Allergy; Sinus; Emotions; Laxative; Raw Lung; Candida Yeast (Natra-Bio); Allergy; or, Sinusitis (Medicine from Nature).

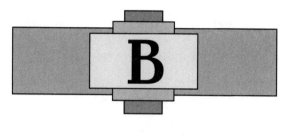

BACKACHE

Backaches are caused by a number of different situations such as a strain or injury from overexercising, lifting, or moving improperly, an accident, poor posture, poor back support, a slipped or ruptured disc, sluggish bowels, kidney problems, emotional stress, and even pregnancy. The problem can be sudden and short lived as in a muscle spasm due to incorrect lifting or the pain may be more persistent.

Begin by checking your posture. See if your shoes are giving you good support; you may need some arch supports or other kinds of inserts. Inspect the area where you work. How you move and sit during the day can impact back soreness. For example, if you hunch over a desk or sit at a keyboard for eight hours without adequate stretching, this can stress your back. Watch how you move to see if you are stressing your back or perhaps you are lifting objects improperly. Inspect your bed. Sometimes the mattress and box springs are sagging and not supporting the body properly. Avoid sofas and chairs that are overstuffed or soft as they do not give good back support.

Check to see if you are drinking enough water throughout the day. If you are not, this may stress the kidneys that lay against the lower back causing back pain. Insufficient water intake can also promote constipation. Eat a sound diet as your back relies on certain nutrients such as calcium to keep it strong.

In addition to the suggested remedies, you might try chiropractic adjustments or therapeutic massages. However, if none of these remedies help, be sure to see a medical doctor for a complete check-up.

KITCHEN REMEDIES

Castor Oil–It is best when this oil is applied warm or use a low, soothing heat source such as a heating pad. This breaks up congested areas in the back and soothes soreness and aches.

Olive Oil–Apply directly to the area of the back that hurts. For best results warm the oil. This tones and soothes the muscles and organs in the back area.

Cranberry Juice–Mix 2 ounces of juice in 2 ounces of water and drink 3-4 times daily. Cranberry juice helps cleanse and strengthen the kidneys.

Parsley Tea–Cut up a handful of parsley and steep in a quart of water for 45 minutes. Strain and cool. Drink half that day and the other half the next day 4 ounces at a time. You can repeat this procedure once a week or for a month for a good cleansing of the kidneys.

> **WARNING:**   Very large doses of parsley leaf may cause nerve damage, bleeding in the gut, liver damage, and abortion.

Prunes–This fruit is not only soothing, but also aids bowel movements thereby taking the pressure off of the low or mid back. Make a juice by soaking the prunes overnight in lemon water. Strain and drink 2-3 times a day, or, drink 3-4 ounces of warm prune juice diluted in equal amounts of water in the morning or at night.

Spikenard–This is a good spice for general backaches and great for easier childbirth. Make a tea.

SINGLE HERBAL REMEDIES

Queen of the Meadow–The aspirin-like substance in this herb helps it relieve pain in the joints. Make a tea or put 10-20 drops of the tincture/extract in juice. Drink 2-3 times a day.

Chaparral–Great for chronic back problems because of its deep cleansing of the muscles and tissue walls. Chaparral is a strong antioxidant and is high in protein and potassium which helps to tone and rebuild the tissues. Make a tea.

Juniper Berries–Assists the joints especially in cases of arthritis. It works equally well when combined with gravel root or Queen of the Meadow for lumbago and sciatica problems. Taking 3 drops of the oil 3-4 times daily in a little juice is very effective. It can be used as a fomentation for pain in the muscles or joints.

WARNING: Do not use juniper if you have any kidney disease or are pregnant without physician supervision.

Wintergreen Oil–The aspirin-like compound in this oil allows it to relieve the pain of rheumatism, sciatica, lumbago, stiff and swollen joints, bruises, sprains, and torn ligaments. Mix 1-2 teaspoons in a pint of warm olive oil or glycerine (you may reduce the amount made depending on amount of liniment needed). Mix well before using and apply to painful area 1-2 times a day. You can also apply heat from hot towels or a heating pad to aid penetration.

Liniment Formula–Mix 1-2 teaspoons of myrrh tincture, 1 teaspoon of goldenseal, 1/2 teaspoon of cayenne in a 1 quart of rubbing alcohol (70%). Or, 2 ounces or 2 capsules of powdered myrrh, 1 ounce or 1 capsule of powdered goldenseal and 1/2 ounce or 1/2 capsule of cayenne pepper in a quart of rubbing alcohol. Prickly ash may be added using 1 teaspoon of tincture, 2 capsules, or 2 ounces of powdered for chronic problems. Mix well and let it stand for seven days, shaking well daily. On the 8th day strain and throw out any residue. Great relief for various aches and pains.

OTHER NATURAL TREATMENTS

Soak Bath–A great relaxing and soothing tonic for an aching back and the whole body. As usual you can add recommended herbs or 1-2 cups of Epsom salts or 1 cup of aloe vera, apple cider vinegar, or baking soda.

Vitamin E (200-400 IU)–Vitamin E improves blood circulation. Because of its antioxidant properties it helps to protect tissues, and the muscles, from damage by free radical molecules. These molecules are created by normal physiological processes. Take 1 capsule 2 times daily. I have seen relief in a few hours when using this vitamin.

> **WARNING:** Avoid Vitamin E supplementation if you are taking blood thinning medication or if you have liver disease. Do not take more than 400 IU of vitamin E for an extended period of time unless under the guidance of a trained professional.

COMMERCIALLY PREPARED HERBAL REMEDIES

Herbs: Kalmin (This antispasmodic tincture can be both taken and rubbed on the area); BF&C (capsules and ointment); KB (for kidney and bladder); Ex-Stress; Naturalax 2; Change-O-Life or Fem-Mend (for female pain) (Nature's Way); Rescue Remedy (Bach); Vegetable Calcium (Schiff's); or, liquid trace mineral (Take 1-2 teaspoons 2-3 times daily in juice. Also moisten a cloth with liquid mineral and lay across the back area for relief covering it with a hot towel or heating pad for 2-5 minutes, when necessary, 1-2 times daily as need.). In addition, there are various natural heat balms and sports injury ointments available for backaches.

Homeopathic: Raw Kidney; Neuralgic Pain; Injuries; Laxative; Emotional; Detoxification; Menstrual; Menopause (Natra-Bio); Injury and Backache (Medicine from Nature), or, Sciatica (Biological Homeopathic Industries).

Note: Liniments or other external remedies containing essential oils will antidote homeopathic remedies.

BEDSORES

Bedsores result from both internal and external causes. Internally, if a patient with no or little sense of pain is lying or sitting for long periods, he doesn't have the feedback he needs to move when his body becomes sore. As a result, the continued pressure (external cause) on a specific area of the body where bones are not sufficiently padded by fat or muscle creates a bed sore. Poor circulation due to immobility contributes to this problem. Infection, anemia, malnutrition, and moist and wrinkled bed clothes make the problem worse.

During the first stage of a bedsore, also called a decubitus ulcer, the skin becomes red. As the condition progresses, the area turns tender and warm, with blisters or general skin irritation. In the worse case scenario, the bedsore can become necrotic all the way through to the fat, muscle, and even bone.

ACTION

Prevention is the best medicine, especially for bedsores. Change body positions every two hours, rolling over to the right or left side of the body or sitting up. Use an "egg carton" mattress in the bed as a cushion to relieve pressure and to aid in air and blood circulation. Air this mat out regularly. Sponge-rubber mattresses, water mattresses, air-filled alternating-pressure mattresses, or even a water bed also help to alleviate excess pressure on sore points. Change bed clothes often, making sure sheets are dry, clean, and wrinkle-free. Inspect skin frequently, especially bony pressure points.

If bedsores have already occurred, wash and clean them with water and a natural soap everyday. Follow this with a natural disinfectant. Keep the person clean and dry, toweling well after baths and sponging skin during hot weather. A well balanced diet is essential. Make sure protein levels are high as this nutrient is vital for tissue repair. Encourage fluid intake, particularly water. To promote blood circulation, passive exercise of the affected areas (you move the body part) or active exercise are helpful. Assist the person in walking around if possible.

KITCHEN REMEDIES

Aloe Vera–Works as a soothing healer of sores and as an antiseptic. Cut a piece of the plant and apply it directly to the worse bedsores several times daily, or, slice a piece lengthwise and bandage or tape it to the infected area. You can use a fresh slice 1-2 times per day or overnight as needed. Aloe vera gel from the health food store works well too.

If you have plenty of aloe vera plants you can make an inexpensive aloe juice by dropping a large amount, like cut celery, of the plant into your blender with blades covered with water and processing on a high speed for a few seconds. Gently apply the amount needed to the bed sores. Refrigerate the remainder in a container with a tight lid if you cannot store the juice in cool room. Keeps for several days. Add less water or glycerin to make a salve. If the aloe vera mixture has been refrigerated, then warm up to baby bottle temperature before applying with a cotton cloth (don't reuse the cloth after an application) or applicator. An easy way to apply the juice is to use a plant sprayer or atomizer. For adults about 1-2 tablespoons to 1-2 ounces straight aloe vera juice in a little juice several times daily is very helpful.

Apple Cider Vinegar–Apply vinegar to the bedsore like a lotion using clean hands, cotton swabs, or a plant sprayer. The vinegar is a soothing healer and an antiseptic.

Castor, Olive, and Wheat Germ Oils–This is a three-oil massage used by most herbalists. The first two days the person should be lightly massaged with warm or room temperature castor oil, using a clockwise circular motion from the top of the head to the bottom of the feet, always moving towards the heart. The next two days use warm or room temperature olive oil, and the last two days of the week use warm or room temperature wheat germ oil. The castor oil cleans and flushes the skin, while the olive oil feeds and rebuilds the muscles and skin, and the wheat germ oil, high in vitamin E, rejuvenates the body. If you have only olive or wheat germ oil on hand, apply either of them directly to the bedsores. In addition, take 1 teaspoon 1-2 times daily of either oil with a juice chaser or in a little food for internal healing.

Garlic and Onions or Cabbage and Potato–Chop or dice either combination of vegetables for a poultice on the bedsores. Be sure to apply a little vegetable or olive oil on the skin to protect it before applying the poultice. Any of these vegetables act as an antiseptic.

Honey–Lightly rub or spray this soothing and antiseptic remedy on the bedsores.

> **WARNING:** Do not apply too often if you are a diabetic.

Witch Hazel–Apply this astringent to the infected area 3-4 times daily. Use fomentation on worse areas by applying warm liquid with a cloth or directly to the affected area. Keep moist by adding the liquid to the cloth or redampen cloth by immersion and reapply.

Corn Starch–Dust the bedsores with a powder puff or cotton ball. If the corn starch does not stick, then mix with a little warm water or vegetable oil to make a paste. Performs as an antiseptic and soothing healer.

SINGLE HERBAL REMEDIES

Any of the liquid herbal remedies listed below can be applied to the bedsores with a plant sprayer or atomizer. Warm up the remedy to a baby bottle temperature before applying for the comfort of the patient.

Black Walnut–Pulls out the infection as well as heals the bedsores. Apply to the bedsores and make a tea.

Myrrh–This is a great healing lotion. Apply directly to area undiluted as a fomentation. Take as a tea as well.

Pau d'Arco–You can use this antiseptic remedy as a tea, fomentation, or as a spray.

Red Clover–Use to make a warm tea, a spray or a fomentation to cleanse the blood and heal wounds.

Slippery Elm - The tincture form is easiest to apply for a an anti-inflammatory and a soothing healer to the bedsores. To foment apply warm liquid with a cloth or directly to the affected area. Also take as a tea. Great food for the body while confined or sick. Can also be used in food as a gruel like oatmeal.

OTHER NATURAL TREATMENTS

Vitamin E and/or A–Apply 200-400 IU of E and/or 5,000 IU of A to the bedsores as needed. Just puncture the capsule or get the bottles of liquid for larger areas. The person can also take 1 capsule 1-2 times daily of both. Either vitamin soothes and heals.

> **WARNING:**   Large doses of vitamin E may interfere with blood clotting. If you are on blood thinning medication or have liver disease, avoid using this vitamin. Don't take more than 50,000 IU of vitamin A daily unless under the guidance of a professional.

COMMERCIALLY PREPARED HERBAL REMEDIES

Herbs: Comfrey, Chickweed, or BF&C (feeds the bone, flesh, joints, and cartilage) ointment; AKN-Skin Care (take and apply as a healing paste or poultice to area several times daily); Echinacea Combination (anti-infection extract); Cal-Silica (A natural calcium to soothe the nerves.); Myrrh-Golden Seal Plus or Root (antibiotic and antiseptic) (Nature's Way); or, liquid trace mineral (A great healer and soother when used on a moistened cloth or cotton and applied to the bedsores several times daily as needed).

Homeopathic: Take 5 Silica 12x tablets 3 times daily. Also, can apply directly to the bed sores, but if too sore mix in a little warm water and apply by cotton or spray several times daily. Also try Injuries; Fever; Neuralgic Pains; Candida Yeast; or, Detoxification (Natra-Bio.).

BITES AND STINGS

Insects and animals sometimes bite or sting us out of fear or by accident. These bites and stings commonly come from bees, wasps, dogs, cats, snakes, gnats, deer flies, chiggers, sand flies, fleas, ticks, mites, spiders, scorpions, caterpillars, mosquitoes, Gila monsters, lizards, jelly fish, or man-o-wars. Depending on the animal, the sting or bite may cause mild to high fever, nausea, dizziness, swelling, pain, a metallic or rubbery taste in the mouth, numbness or tingling around the mouth, headache, thirst, blurred vision, skin rash, weakness, itching, shortness of breath, anxiety, vomiting, or other symptoms.

Hydrophobia, a term used to describe rabies in humans, usually results from a bite from a rabid dog or other animal. This disease can take anywhere from 10 days to over a year to manifest. Early symptoms include restlessness, melancholy, loss of sleep, fever, and malaise. These feelings develop as a tightness around throat and difficulty in swallowing become apparent. The person begins to salivate excessively and although she or he has a great thirst, cannot drink. Convulsions, severe difficulty in breathing and choking on saliva can occur in three to 10 days. Death is a result of exhaustion, paralysis, and asphyxiation.

> **WARNING:** For bad bites or stings, compress or tie off vein above the wound, but not too tight, with a belt, rope, etc. Then apply herbs to neutralize the poisons while seeking immediate medical help. If you've been bitten by a wild animal or dog, see your physician about the possibility of rabies. If you're bitten by a cat or another person and the skin is broken, see your doctor.

ACTION

For stings remove stinger by scraping the stinger with a credit card or your nail. Do not try to pull the stinger out with tweezers as this may release more poison into your system. Wash out the wound with a natural soap and water, apply a natural disinfectant and apply the following suggested remedies immediately. Repeat as needed.

For bites wash area immediately with a natural disinfectant. Take suggested remedies either internally or apply herbs, especially burdock, as a poultice or fomentation to the bite. Again, it is important to check with a doctor right away in cases of very bad bites. If the bite is from a rabid animal, trap it or see where the animal went, then call the police and an animal shelter to come and get the animal.

KITCHEN REMEDIES

Aloe Vera–Cut a piece of the plant and apply directly to the area several times daily, or slice the piece length wise and band-aid or tape it to the bite or sting. You can use a fresh slice 1-2 times per day or overnight as needed. If you have plenty of aloe vera plants you can make inexpensive aloe juice by dropping a large amount, like cut celery, of the plant into your blender with the blades covered with water, processing on high speed for a few seconds. Take the amount needed, then store refrigerated in a container with a tight lid. Keeps for several days. Add less water or glycerin to make a paste and apply to the bite or sting.

Apple Cider Vinegar–Mix a 1/4 teaspoon of this antiseptic in a cup of water and drink every 1-2 hours as need. You can also apply apple cider vinegar directly to the bite or sting several times a day.

Baking Soda–Ingest slowly 1/4 teaspoon in 4 ounces of warm water every 1-2 hours as needed. Mix it with a little water and apply, or soak the area as needed. Baking soda neutralizes most of the acids from bites and stings. **WARNING:** Unless a doctor supervises, do not administer to children under 5 years old. Don't take more than 1/2 tsp. 8 times a day if you're under 60 years old or 1/2 tsp. 4 times a day if you're over 60 in a 24-hour period. Don't take this maximum dose for more than 2 weeks. Don't use baking soda if you're on a sodium-restricted diet.

Meat Tenderizer–Mix water with the meat tenderizer to make a paste, then apply to the bite or sting. The natural papain in meat tenderizers neutralizes the poison.

Butter and/or Salt–Using either one of these antiseptics is good for non-poisonous bites and stings. Apply butter directly to area. When using salt slightly moisten it with water before applying.

Lemon–For faster results from this antiseptic fresh lemons are best. Take 1/2 teaspoon in a cup of water every 1-2 hours as needed and lightly apply to the sting or bite.

Garlic or Onion–You can use fresh, powdered, flakes, crushed, or diced garlic or onion. Mix either antiseptic vegetable in little vegetable oil and apply to the bite or sting. You can also take a little of the garlic in a glass of juice. The onion draws out the poison and the stinger, while garlic is a natural antiseptic.

Basil–This remedy is a great support for shock or a collapse and it is a strong antispasmodic. In addition, it draws out the poisons from insect, snake, and dog bites. Make a tea or use as a fomentation.

Mayonnaise–Spread this antacid over the sting or bite. If you have a mayonnaise made from either safflower or apple cider vinegar, both are very good antiseptics. If not, you can add 1 teaspoon safflower oil or apple cider vinegar to 1/2 cup of mayonnaise.

Witch Hazel–Apply some witch hazel directly to sting or bite to help stop any bleeding

SINGLE HERBAL REMEDIES

Burdock–Helps heal lesions created by an insect, rabid dog and other animal bite. Use as a fomentation.

Echinacea–Cleanses blood stream of poisons and is especially good for spider, snake, and insect bites. This remedy is used by Sioux Indians for snake bites and rabies (hydrophobia). Make a tea or use as a fomentation.

Skullcap (Mad Dog Weed) or Valerian Root–These nervines work well as tonics for the nerves and for convulsions. They are harmless to the body's system even if taken in large doses for severe cases. If it is not stated on the bottle then add 10-20 drops of the tincture or extract or 3-5 drops of the herbal oil in a cup of hot water, water at room temperature or fruit juice. Stir the mixture and drink it 2-3 times daily.

White Oak Bark–A great astringent and neutralizer of poisons, this herb works well for insects and snake bites. Make a tea.

OTHER NATURAL TREATMENTS

Vitamin A (5,000 IU) and D (400 IU)–If you are bitten by sand worms this remedy works very well, however, you may use it for other kinds of bites. Take 1 capsule or tablet 2 times daily. You may also grind or smash either vitamin up, add a little water or vegetable oil to make a paste and apply directly to the bite or sting. If you have perles, puncture them and apply directly. **WARNING:** Both Vitamins A and D are potentially toxic if taken in very large amount for long periods of time. Use this treatment temporarily.

Vitamin E (400 IU)–This is especially good for chigger and nonpoisonous bites. Take 1 capsule 2 times daily. You may puncture a perle and apply directly on the bite. **WARNING:** Avoid vitamin E supplementation if you are taking blood thinning medication or if you have liver disease. Don't take more than 400 I.U.s of vitamin E for any length of time unless under the guidance of a physician.

COMMERCIALLY PREPARED HERBAL REMEDIES

Herbs: BF&C (Rebuilds bone, flesh and cartilage.); Comfrey, Chickweed or Black ointment; Kalmin (anti-spasmodic tincture); Red Clover Combination (capsules or syrup purifies blood stream) (Nature's Way); Rescue Remedy (for shock and trauma)(Bach); or, liquid trace mineral (A great healing disinfectant that can be applied directly with a piece of cotton as needed.).

Homeopathic: Insect Bites, Injuries, Detoxification (Natra-Bio); or, SssstingStop (Soothing repellent and bug gel.) (Boericke & Tafel).

BLEEDING

Bleeding can occur for numerous reasons in all parts of the body: external injuries such as cuts, internal bleeding like hemorrhoids, or even normal body functions such as a menstrual period. At times, bleeding will not be serious like a mild nose bleed or blood in your stools due to straining bowel movements. Other times, the situation will be more urgent. You may be bleeding and not even know it. Black, tarry stools indicate bleeding high in your colon.

Excessive menstrual flow can also be a problem (see "Menstrual Problems"). It is normal for a woman to pass blood, called lochia, after childbirth. However, when this flow becomes excessive something is wrong. This can range from a cut of the cervix or uterus to a retained placenta. These situations are usually detected and taken care of shortly after childbirth. However, there are rare instances where a small portion of a placenta remains in the womb after delivery. If a woman begins to hemorrhage after childbirth, whatever the reason, call her doctor immediately.

When too much blood is lost, either suddenly or over a long period of time, weakness, shock, anemia, and a drop in blood pressure may result. While this section will address bleeding in general, see other parts of this book for specific problems.

There are three types of bleeding wounds. Knowing which kind you're dealing with will help determine your first aid treatment. When bleeding is from a severed or badly cut artery, bright red, oxygen-rich blood spurts from the wound. Arterial blood comes directly from the heart and spurts at each heartbeat.

A vein has been cut when the blood is dark red and flows in a steady stream. Carbon dioxide, less oxygen, and waste products cause this dark red color. Surface cuts usually injure only the capillaries, or small blood vessels. Relatively little blood is lost in these cases. Usually direct pressure with a compress over the wound will cause the formation of a clot and stop the bleeding. The greatest threat when capillaries are damaged is when large skin surface is involved, then infection is a concern.

> **WARNING:** If this is a serious wound with a lot of bleeding, get to a doctor soon as possible. Loss of more than one quart of blood can be life threatening. A severed artery or serious wound may require stitches. Excessive vaginal bleeding after childbirth needs a doctor's attention immediately.

ACTION

If bleeding is from a small wound or cut, let it bleed a little to clean itself out. Then wash the wound with water and apply a natural disinfectant. Because many of the remedies listed in this section stop simple bleeding, prevent infections, and seal and heal the wound, apply them before you bandage the wound.

To stop the bleeding, apply direct pressure (Figures 1-4). Place a gauze or clean cloth over the bleeding point and apply firm pressure until a covering bandage is applied. The knot of the covering bandage should be tied over the wound in such a way that direct pressure is applied. If bleeding continues after the bandage has been put on, then not enough pressure has been applied. Then use the hand to put more pressure on the wound over the bandage, or apply a second bandage. Whatever you do, **do not** remove the original dressing.

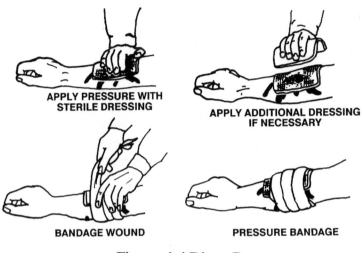

APPLY PRESSURE WITH
STERILE DRESSING

APPLY ADDITIONAL DRESSING
IF NECESSARY

BANDAGE WOUND

PRESSURE BANDAGE

Figures 1-4 Direct Pressure

If the wound needs bandaging, see the recommended techniques in Figures 5-16. Not every area of the body that may need bandaging is covered; however, what is shown may be easily adapted to any immediate situation. When bandaging the wound be sure that the bandage is snug, but not too tight as it may damage the surrounding tissue or interfere with the blood supply, especially if swelling occurs. On the other hand, a bandage too loose may slip off the wound. Remember when bandaging arms or legs to leave the tips of the fingers or toes uncovered where possible so that any interference with circulation can be detected. To tie off the bandage use a square knot so that the knot will not come loose.

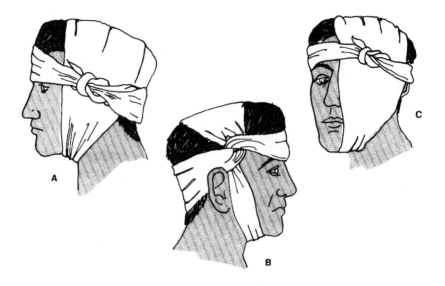

Figure 5-7 Head Bandaging

- Apply the pad of a bandage compress over the wound.
- Carry one end under the chin, and the other over the top of the head.
- Cross at the temple in front of the ear on the side opposite the injury.
- Bring one end around the front of the head and the other end low around the back of the head.
- Tie on or near the compress pad.
- Cover the compress with a cravat bandage applied in the same manner.

If the wound is on the cheek or the front of the face, cross the bandage compress and cravat bandage behind the ear, on the side opposite the injury; bring the ends around the forehead and back of the head, and tie.

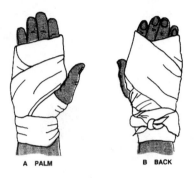

A PALM   B BACK

Figure 8-9 Hand Bandage

To dress a wound of the palm or back of the hand, proceed as follows:

- Apply the pad of a bandage compress over the wound.
- Pass the ends several times around the hand and wrist.
- Tie over the pad.
- Place the center of a cravat bandage over the pad.
- Cross the ends at the opposite side of the hand.
- Pass one end around the little finger side of the hand.
- Pass the other ends and continue around the wrist, crossing at the back of the wrist.
- Cross the ends and continue around the wrist, crossing at the back of the wrist.
- Cross again at the inside of the wrist.
- Tie at the back of the wrist.
- Place the forearm and hand in a triangular bandage sling.

Finger and End of Finger

To dress a wound of the finger, proceed as follows:

- Apply the pad of a small bandage compress over the wound
- Pass the ends several times around the finger and tie over the pad.

- A small adhesive compress may be used instead of a bandage compress for a wound of the finger or a wound on the end of the finger. A bent finger should be dressed bent and not fully extended.
- If more than one finger is injured, cover with an open triangle bandage as for extensive wounds of the hand.

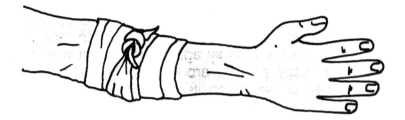

Figure 10 Forearm Bandage

To bandage wounds of the arm, forearm, and wrist, proceed as follows:

- Apply the pad of a sterile bandage compress over the wound.
- Pass the ends several times around the arm and tie them over the pad.
- Place the center of a cravat bandage over the pad.
- Pass the ends around the arm, cross them, continue around the arm and tie over the pad (Figure 10).
- Place the forearm and hand in a triangular sling.

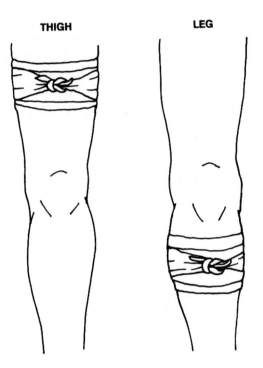

Figures 11-12 Thigh and Leg Bandage

To tie a bandage for a wound of the thigh or leg, proceed as follows:

- Apply the pad of a bandage compress over the wound.
- Pass the ends around the injured part and tie over the pad.
- Place the center of a cravat bandage over the compress, pass the ends around the injured part, cross them, bring them around again, and tie over the pad.

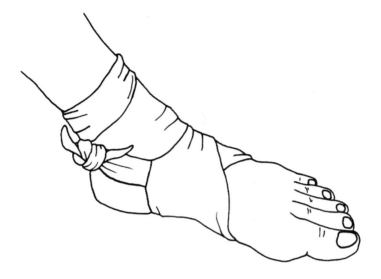

Figure 13 Ankle Bandage

To dress a wound of the ankle, proceed as follows:

- Apply the pad of bandage compress to the wound.
- Carry the ends to the top of the instep and cross.
- Carry the ends around the bottom of the foot and cross over the instep again.
- Pass the ends around the ankle and tie over the pad.
- Place the center of a cravat bandage over the compress.
- Carry the ends to the top of the instep, cross.
- Cross the ends under the foot, bring back to the top of the instep and cross.
- Carry the ends around the ankle and tie over the pad.

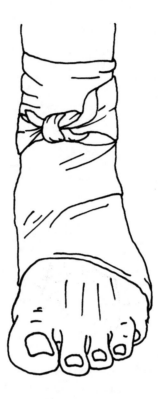

Figure 14 Foot Bandage

To dress a wound of the foot proceed as follows:

- Apply the pad of a bandage compress to the wound.
- Carry the ends around the foot and ankle.
- Tie over the pad.
- Place the center of a cravat bandage over the compress.
- Carry the ends around the foot and ankle, ending in tie as near the front of the ankle as possible.

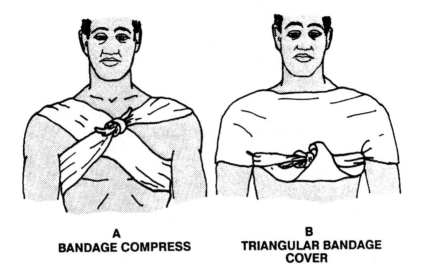

A
BANDAGE COMPRESS

B
TRIANGULAR BANDAGE
COVER

Figures 15-16 Chest Bandage

To dress around on the chest or back between the shoulder blades, proceed as follows:

- Place the pad of the compress over the wound so that the ends are diagonally across the chest or back.
- Carry one end over the shoulder and under the armpit. Carry the other end under the armpit and over the shoulder,. Tie the ends over the compress.

Cover the compress and chest or back with a triangular bandage as follows:

- Place the center of the base at the lower part of the neck.
- Allow the apex to drop down over the chest or back, as appropriate.
- Carry the ends over the shoulders and under the armpits to the center of the chest or back.
- Tie with the apex below the knot.
- Turn the apex up and tuck it over the knot.

Back, Chest, Abdomen, or Side

To tie a bandage for the back, chest, abdomen, or side, proceed as follow:

- Apply the pad of a sterile bandage compress or sterile gauze over the wound. If a sterile bandage compress is used, take the ends around the body (one end across the back and the other across the abdomen or chest and tie on the side.)
- Cover with a proper size cravat bandage by placing the center of the bandage on the side nearest the injury.
- Take the ends across the back and abdomen or chest and tie on the opposite side.

Note: If air is being sucked into the lungs through a wound in the chest, cover the wound at once with a nonporous material (plastic wrap, wax paper, or your hand). Then dress the wound. Transport to a medical facility immediately.

KITCHEN REMEDIES

Cayenne–The powder is the best to quickly coagulate the blood and seal the wound. It's even quicker than a tincture. Apply directly to the bleeding area. You can also take a 1/4 teaspoon of the powder in water or juice. For a nose bleed, either sniff cayenne powder up the nose through a straw or from some in the hand. For bleeding gums hold the aforementioned solution in the mouth or pack powder in the gum area where it is bleeding. Discontinue use if the cayenne irritates or burns your skin. You can also use cayenne oil from the health food store.

Sage–Apply sage leaves or powder directly to bleeding area. You can sniff sage up the nose or pack gums with it. Make a thick tea which may also be held in the mouth and used as drops for the nose.

Onion–Chopped, diced, or squeezed for its juice, the onion disinfects the wound. Mix the onion with a little apple cider vinegar. Use for nose bleeds by snuffing drops up the nose with an eye dropper or holding solution in the mouth for bleeding gum. (**Note:** If your gums chronically bleed, see your dentist.)

Cranberry–Drinking cranberry juice is the best and it can be applied directly to the wound working as an antiseptic and a mild coagulant.

Witch Hazel–Use externally for cuts and wounds as a mild coagulant. However, this is also good for the gums and nose.

Cobwebs–This ancient remedy still works so don't be squeamish. It binds the cut and helps the blood to dry faster.

SINGLE HERBAL REMEDIES

Alfalfa–Since alfalfa is high in vitamin K, it helps to clot the blood. You can use as a tea or as a fomentation. If removing the cloth would open the wound, just remoisten the cloth and leave on until it can come loose without tearing the area.

Aloe Vera–Either the gel or concentrated liquid is great for healing as a natural antibiotic and infection fighter and relieves pain. Apply directly with a moistened cotton then band-aid or tape it to the wound. You can also soak the cut in the liquid.

Shepherd's Purse–A general, all purpose remedy particularly good for bleeding problems, externally as well as internally. Make a tea.

White Oak Bark–This is an all purpose remedy which works great for a bleeding rectum, nose, gums, and veins. Make a tea. For bleeding bowels, also take in a total of 1 pint of herbal tea in the rectum as an implant. This can be done a few times a week to heal and strengthen. If there is unusual vaginal bleeding you may use the implant to stop the bleeding. (See "Menstrual problems.")

Red Raspberry–For bleeding and recovery after childbirth, red raspberry is renowned for toning and healing the uterus. Best used as a tea with a little honey. Drink every 2 hours.

Black Cohosh–This extract helps normalize the female hormones and reproductive system after pregnancy, and eases after pains. Use as a tea. Drink every 1-2 hours.

OTHER NATURAL TREATMENTS

Vitamin K–Helps the blood clot. Use the water-soluble form. Take 2 capsules daily.

COMMERCIALLY PREPARED HERBAL REMEDIES

Herbs: Comfrey or BF&C (ointments or capsules may be taken and use a fomentation by applying warm ointment or mixing capsules in warm oil with a cloth or directly to the affected area. Keep moist by adding the ointment or mixture to the cloth or redampen cloth by immersion and reapply.); Myrrh-Goldenseal Plus capsules (great infection fighters); Rescue Remedy (for shock and trauma) (Bach); or, liquid trace mineral (Great for fighting infections and stops bleeding. Moisten cloth or cotton with liquid mineral and apply several times daily as needed.)

Homeopathic: Injuries; Hemorrhoids; or, Menstrual (Natra-Bio); or, Bleeding (Biological Homeopathic Industries).

BLISTERS

Blisters, a tender, irritated skin condition, are usually formed from rubbing, scraping, or friction on the feet or toes from new shoes and on the hands from doing manual labor like digging, and burns from hot pots, matches, or lit cigarettes.

ACTION

Wash the blisters with a natural soap and then use a natural disinfectant. Make physical adjustments to help eliminate the cause of the blisters like not wearing new shoes for too long or using gloves for manual labor. Apply remedy and put a bandage over the area for protection.

KITCHEN REMEDIES

Corn Starch–Mix the corn starch, which acts like an antiseptic and soothes, with a little warm water or vegetable oil and spread over area. Cover with a bandage if needed.

Honey or Apple Cider Vinegar–Both remedies fight bacteria in the blister. Mix a little together or use separately and spread over blister. Apply a bandage if needed.

Olive or Wheat Germ Oil–Rub either oil lightly over the blister and apply a bandage. The oils heal and soothe the skin.

SINGLE HERBAL REMEDIES

Dandelion–Use the juice from a freshly picked flower stem to rub over the blister. Or, you may pick a bunch of flower stems and make a poultice. Dandelions purify the blood and improve circulation moving clean blood through the body to help healing. Dandelion ointment from a health food store can also be applied to the blister or use the tincture to make a fomentation.

Aloe Vera–Spread the gel, which is a natural infection fighter, carefully over the blistered area, then cover with gauze or a bandage. Aloe vera also soothes the pain.

Myrrh–Apply a few drops on the blister or use the ointment as an infection fighter for blisters.

Comfrey or Chickweed–Use either or both of these as wound healers. Make a fomentation. You may also use the ointment of either remedy.

OTHER NATURAL TREATMENTS

Vitamin A and E–Puncture a perle and apply the liquid directly on the blister, or smash a tablet up mixing with a little water or oil then apply to area. Either vitamin soothes the pain and acts as an anti-oxygenate to speed healing.

COMMERCIALLY PREPARED HERBAL REMEDIES

Herbs: BF&C (Rebuilds bones, flesh, and cartilage.) Echinacea-Golden Seal Root extract or Pau d'Arco Bark extract (good infection fighters.); or, Liquid Trace Mineral (Great for fighting infections and stops bleeding. Moisten cloth or cotton with liquid mineral and apply several times daily as needed.)

Homeopathic: Injuries; Fever; or, Pain (Natra-Bio); Injury & Backache (Medicine from Nature).

BLOOD POISONING

Blood poisoning, also called bacteremia, is caused by bacteria infecting the blood system. This condition can be caused by surgical intervention, a medically implanted device in a blood vessel or a urethral catheter. Sometimes a blood infection arises from an infection in another part of the body such as the lungs, gut, joints, bones, or skin. Wounds can lead to septicemia. (See "Bleeding.")

Usually bacteremia is temporary and may not even be detected. In cases where symptoms occur, this condition is called septicemia. The onset of chills are usual, followed by profuse perspiration, rapid pulse and breathing, fever, depression or an anxious expression, nausea, vomiting, and diarrhea. Skin eruptions may appear such as small, red dots, blisters, or red streaks that feel hot to the touch.

> **WARNING:** Call a doctor if these symptoms appear. Untreated septicemia can have severe consequences.

ACTION

Select a listed remedy to ingest and apply a remedy to the red streak on the arm or leg. Keep the person warm and calm while awaiting professional medical help. Give 4-6 ounces of water every hour to move the toxins out of the body. While you may use the following home treatments, don't put off getting proper medical attention.

KITCHEN REMEDIES

Cayenne Pepper–Mix 1/4 teaspoon of the cayenne, a natural antiseptic, in water or a juice. Drink it down and repeat as needed. You may also use cayenne for a poultice. Mix the pepper to form a paste with warm or hot water, warm vegetable or wheat germ oil. Apply the paste directly to the area or place inside a cloth (cotton, wool, or flannel) then place over infected area.

Apple Cider Vinegar–This natural disinfectant applied directly to a wound, is an internal cleanser. For adults take 1 teaspoon in water or apple juice 2-4 times a day.

Garlic or Onion–Use these vegetables as an antiseptic poultice.

Raisins–Eat a hand full several times a day to cleanse the blood and as an antiseptic. My grandparents had me do this for boils when I was young. It never failed.

SINGLE HERBAL REMEDIES

Echinacea–King of the blood purifiers, this herb is especially good for swelling. In severe cases use 20-30 drops in a cup of warm water or 2 capsules every 2 hours. Also apply echinacea directly to streaks on legs as a fomentation.

Goldenseal–Acts as a cleanser and infection fighter. Make a tea.

Plantain–Reduces swelling and pain, red streaking, and may prevent amputation. For a severe condition use 20-30 drops or 2 capsules, in a of cup strong tea every 2 hours.

Marshmallow–Use as an external aid to draw out the poisons and soothe. Works great when you can mix with a little cayenne in it. Apply warm liquid with a cloth or directly to the affected area. Keep moist by adding the liquid to the cloth or redampen the cloth by immersion and reapply.

Red Clover–Purifies the blood stream. For acute conditions take 20-30 drops or 2 capsules, in a cup of strong tea every 2 hours.

OTHER NATURAL TREATMENTS

Soak Bath–A great drawing and cleansing tonic for the whole body. The heat expands the skin and inner body tissue drawing the toxins to the skin's surface and into the water. While filling the tub with hot water add 1-2 cups of Epsom salt. You may also soak just the feet by adding 1/2-1 cup of Epsom salt to pan or container.

Enema–This pulls out lower bowel poisons. It is best to do this when the first signs of blood poisoning appear. Mix 1 teaspoon of baking soda or the juice of 1/2 of a **fresh** lemon with seeds strained, into a bag of warm distilled or spring water.

COMMERCIALLY PREPARED HERBAL REMEDIES

Herbs: Kalmin (antispasmodic extract); H Formula (Strengthens heart and blood); Red Clover Combination (Cleanses the blood stream.) (Nature's Way); Rescue Remedy (for shock and trauma) (Bach); or, liquid trace mineral (Cleanses blood infections and streaking. Give 1-2 Ounces in about 4-6 ounces of water or juice several times throughout the day as needed.)

Homeopathic: Take 2 Lachesis l2X tablets or 10 drops every 1-2 hours for severe cases. Otherwise about 3-4 times daily. Also try, Injuries; Fever; Nausea; Detoxification; or, Pain (Natra-Bio).

BOILS

Boils were one of the plagues of the Egyptians. A boil, actually an abscess that has developed in a hair follicle, is due to a staphylococcal infection. This infection usually occurs on the face, neck, breasts, or buttocks. They can be very painful if on the fingers, nose, ear, or other part of the body where an underlying structure is attached to the boil. Boils lie just under the skin as a red bump and can develop into a pustule with a white, reddish discharge. They can be very painful, swollen, tender, and reddish.

When boils become a chronic problem it's called furunculosis. A cluster of slowly healing boils under the skin is called a carbuncle. Poor diet and a slow eliminating system sets up the body for boils.

ACTION

Improve your diet by eating more grains, fiber, vegetables, and fruit. Drink more water to flush the toxins from the body through the kidneys, bowels and skin. A hot moist cloth placed over the boil will help it "mature." Once it comes to a head, and only then, you can lance the boil with a disinfected needle. Do this at the base of the boil close to the skin so it will heal better. Sometimes a boil will drain on its own. In either case, disinfect the area afterwards and apply the one of the listed remedies.

Before using the disinfectant and suggested aid, gently wash the boil with a natural soap and water, then apply a natural disinfectant.

KITCHEN REMEDIES

Aloe Vera–Use this natural antibiotic by cutting a piece of the plant and applying it directly to the boil several times daily, or slicing the piece lengthwise and bandage or tape it to the boil. You can use a fresh slice 1-2 times per day or overnight as needed. If you have plenty of aloe vera plants you can make inexpensive aloe juice by dropping a large amount, like cut celery, of the plant into your blender with the blades covered with water, processing on high speed for a few seconds. Take the amount needed, then store refrigerated in a container with a tight lid. This keeps for several days. Add less water or glycerin to make a paste and apply to the boil. Good for healing infections and sores as well as boils.

Apple Cider Vinegar–In 6 ounces of water mix 1-2 teaspoons of apple cider vinegar, an infection fighter, and drink it down. Do this 3-4 times daily. You can dab some of the vinegar directly on the boil. Apple cider vinegar is great for all pus formations. Also works great when mixing 2 quarts of apple cider vinegar and 8 ounces of garlic or onion juice. Shake well before drinking 1 ounce undiluted or in 3-5 ounces of juice 3-4 times daily.

Onions/Garlic–Use fresh onions or garlic either in combination or singularly to make an antiseptic poultice. You can use garlic oil as well. Always apply vegetable oil over the boil before using garlic.

Sage or Rosemary–Take either anti-inflammatory as tea or use as a poultice. Do **not** drink more than 3 cups of tea during a 24 hour period.

Cabbage or Potatoes–Both of these vegetables have great drawing power. Make a poultice using either vegetable separately or in combination.

Figs–Fresh figs are best. Mash them up and apply as a warm poultice to the boil. Figs pull the infections out. Used to heal King Ahab from a "sickness unto death."

Raisins–These are great infection fighters that are high in iron. Eat 2 handfuls a day for 1-2 weeks. Raisins eliminated many severe, painful boils on my legs as a child in a few weeks. This remedy was suggested by my grandmother.

SINGLE HERBAL REMEDIES

Burdock Root–This has no equal. It is the best blood purifier, especially for chronic infections, and skin problems. Make a tea or use as a fomentation.

Echinacea or Pau d'Arco–Both of these are good infection fighters that combat carbuncles and abscesses. Make a tea. Also foment the boil by applying the warm oil or liquid with a cloth or directly onto the affected area.

Red Clover–Cleanses the blood stream. Make a tea.

Sarsaparilla or Sassafras–Both are great skin and blood cleansers. You can either apply directly to the problem area or drink as a tea. As a preventive, drink 1 cup of tea daily or blend in a 50/50 mixture with other herbs.

OTHER NATURAL TREATMENTS

Vitamin A and E–Great for skin problems. Open 1-2 capsules and apply either singularly or both to boil or carbuncle by puncturing the perle. In tablet form smash or grind the tablets adding a little warm water or vegetable oil to make a paste and then apply.

COMMERCIALLY PREPARED HERBAL REMEDIES

Herbs: Kalmin (anti-spasmodic tincture); BF&C; Chickweed or Black ointment and/or capsules (good infection fighter); AKN-Skin Care; Myrrh-Golden Seal Plus (good infection fighter) (Nature's

Way); or, liquid trace mineral (A good infection fighter that rebuilds the overall body systems. Take 1 teaspoon in apple juice 1-2 times daily and moisten cloth or cotton with mineral and apply to the boil several times daily to speed healing.)

Homeopathics: Detoxification; Injuries; or, Raw Liver (Natra-Bio).

BONES

Bone injuries include fractures, bruises, or dislocations. Sometimes this kind of injury can cause severe trauma and be a slow-healing process. Osteoporosis, an affliction usually of the elderly and more often among women, cause bones to become brittle. When this disorder progresses far enough, stepping off a curb or turning in bed is sometimes enough movement to cause a fracture.

Low estrogen levels put post menopausal women at greater risk of developing osteoporosis. Low calcium intake (especially early in life), smoking, lack of exercise, caffeine, and an inadequate diet also promote this potentially debilitating disease.

> **WARNING:** Get medical help immediately if the injury or fall appears severe, especially if the bone has broken through the skin or bleeding. When applying first aid, move the victim as little as possible. This is especially important if the person has spinal injuries.

ACTION

First call for an ambulance. If the person is in a great deal of pain or you suspect a fracture, try not to move him until experienced help arrives. Otherwise, try to immobilize the area with splint-like devices (wood, metal, rolled, or folded newspapers) around the area and tie the splints together with belts, sheets, ropes (see Figures 17-27 for examples on how to do splints). Elevate the affected limbs without disturbing the suspected fractured area. If you suspect a dislocation, splint as above. If skin is broken around the break and the bone is sticking through it (compound fracture) keep the area clean with natural disinfectants and herbal aid.

Do not try to set a fracture. If you suspect a dislocation, do not try to correct the problem. Also see the section on "Bleeding" for additional suggestions. Keep the person as still as possible. Only move the patient if necessary such as a fire. Use the following aids to speed healing.

Splints

Use splints to support, immobilize, and protect parts with injuries such as known or suspected fractures, dislocations, or severe sprains. When in doubt, treat the injury as a fracture and splint it. Splints prevent movement at the area of the injury and at the nearest joints. Splints should immobilize and support the joint or bones above and below the break.

Many types of splints are available commercially. Easily applied and quickly inflated plastic splints give support to injured limbs. Improvised splints may be made from pieces of wood, broom handles, newspapers, heavy cardboard, boards, magazines, or similar firm materials (Figures 17-18).

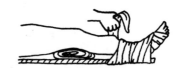

SUPPORT AND SLIDE WELL-PADDED
SPLINT UNDER LEG

PAD SPACES BETWEEN LEG AND SPLINT
AND BANDAGE SECURELY

Figures 17-18 Splinting

Certain guidelines should be followed when splinting:

- Gently remove all clothing from any suspected fracture or dislocation.
- Do not attempt to push bones back through an open wound.
- Do not attempt to straighten any fracture.
- Cover open wounds with a sterile dressing before splinting.

- Pad splints with soft material to prevent excessive pressure on the affected area and to aid in supporting the injured part.
- Pad under all natural arches of the body such as the knee and wrist.
- Support the injured part while splint is being applied.
- Splint firmly, but not so tightly as to interfere with circulation or cause undue pain.
- Support fracture or dislocation before transporting victim.

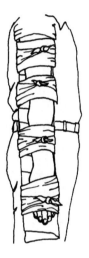

Figure 19 Straight Arm or Elbow Splint

Lower Two-Thirds of Arm, Elbow, Forearm, or Wrist

Take extreme care when dealing with a fractured elbow, as the fracture may cause extensive damage to surrounding tissues, nerves, and blood vessels. Improper care and handling of a fractured elbow could result in a permanent disability. The symptoms of a fractured elbow are as follows:

The first aid for a fractured elbow or arm in a straight position is as follows:

- Do not bend, straighten, or twist the arm in any direction.
- Use a splint long enough to reach from 1 inch below the armpit to 1 inch beyond the tip of the middle finger.

- While the fracture is being supported, pad to conform to the deformity and place splint on the inner side of the arm.
- Place the center of the first cravat bandage on the outside of the arm at the upper end of the splint, cross on the inside of the arm over the splint, pass the ends one or more times around the arm and splint, and tie on the outside.
- Place the centers of the second and third cravat bandages on the arm just above and below the elbow, and apply in a similar manner.
- Center the fourth cravat bandage on the back of the wrist. Pass the ends around and cross on the splint under the wrist, bring one end up around the little finger side. and cross over the back of the hand and down between the forefinger and thumb. Pass the other end up over the thumb, cross it over the back of the hand down around the little finger side, then cross both ends on the splint and tie on top of the hand.
- Tie a fifth cravat bandage around the splint, arm, and body to prevent movement during transportation.

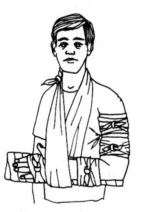

Figure 20 Bent Arm or Elbow Splint

If the arm is bent, immobilize in a bent position by making an L-shaped splint for the forearm and wrist from two pieces of bard 1/4 inch thick and 4 inches wide. One piece should be long enough to extend from 1 inch below the armpit to the point of the elbow and the other long enough to extend from the point of the elbow to 1 inch beyond the end of the middle finger. Immobilize the limb to the splint in the following manner.

- Fasten the boards together securely to form an L-shaped splint.
- Pad the splint.
- While an assistant supports the fracture on both sides of the break apply the splint to the inner side of the arm and forearm after placing the forearm across the chest.
- Use four cravat bandages to hold the splint in place.
- Place the center of the first cravat bandage on the outside of the arm at the upper end of the splint, pass around the arm one or more times, and tie on the arm.
- Place the centers of the second and third cravat bandages on the arm and forearm, respectively, passing around one or more times and tying on the arm.
- Apply the fourth cravat bandage by placing the center of the bandage on the back of the wrist, passing the ends around and crossing on the splint under the wrist. Take one end up around the little finger side, passing over the back of the hand and down between the forefinger and thumb. Pass the other end up over the thumb, and cross it over the back of the hand down around the little finger side; then cross both ends on the splint and tie on top of the hand.
- Place the arm in a cravat bandage sling (Figure 20).

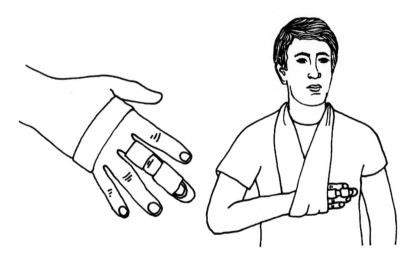

Figures 21-22 Finger Splint

The first aid for a fractured finger is as follows:

- Place a narrow padded splint under the broken finger and palm of the hand.
- Pass a narrow strip of cloth around the splint and palm of the hand; tie over the splint.
- Pass a narrow strip of cloth around the finger and the splint above the fracture; tie over the splint.
- Pass a narrow strip of cloth around the finger and the splint below the fracture; tie over the splint.
- Place the hand in a narrow cravat bandage sling.

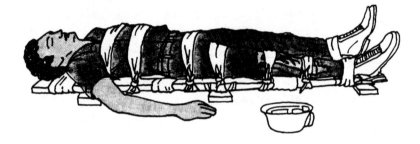

Figure 23 Thigh or Knee Splint

Any improvised splint for the thigh or knee should be long enough to immobilize the hip and the ankle.

If a fracture of the thigh or knee is open, dress the wound. If the fracture is at the knee joint and the limb is not in a straight position, make no attempt to straighten the limb. Splint in line of deformity. Attempts to straighten the limb may increase the possibility of permanent damage. Improvise a way to immobilize the knee as it is found, using padding to fill any space. Use the utility splint stretcher or a similar support to immobilize fractures of the knee or thigh. Before placing the victim on the stretcher, it should be well padded and tested. Additional padding will also be necessary for the natural arches of the body. Raise the victim carefully for placement on the stretcher while the fracture is supported from the underside on both sides of the break.

Apply the splint with bandages. All bandages should be tied on the injured side near the splint.

- Tie the first bandage around the body and splint under the armpits.
- Tie the second around the chest and splint and the third around the hips and splint.
- Tie the fourth and fifth bandages on the injured leg just below the crotch at the thigh and above the knee, respectively, (above and below fracture) and tie on the injured side near the splint.
- Tie the sixth and seventh bandages on the injured leg below the knee and at the ankle.
- An additional bandage at the ankle on the uninjured side may be needed for additional support.
- The victim should be transported on a regular stretcher or stretcher board.

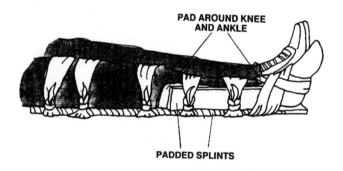

Figure 24 Leg or Ankle Splint

If the fracture is open, dress the wound before splinting. When it is necessary to remove a shoe or boot because of pain from swelling of the ankle or for any other reason, the removal must be carefully done by unlacing or cutting the boot to prevent damage to the ankle. In the absence of severe swelling or bleeding it may be wise to leave the boot on for additional support.

The splint for a fracture of the leg or ankle should reach from against the buttocks to beyond the heel. Place a well-padded splint under the victim while the leg is supported on both sides of the fracture. Tie the bandages on the outer side, near the splint as follows:

- Pass the end of the first bandage around the inner side of the thigh at the groin, pass it over the thigh under the splint, and tie.
- Pass two bandages around the thigh and splint, one at the middle of the thigh and the other just above the knee and tie.
- Place additional padding around the outer part of the leg (Figure 24).
- Pass a fourth bandage around the leg, the padding, and the splint just below the knee and tie; pass a fifth bandage just above or below the fracture and tie (do not tie over the fracture).
- Pass the center of sixth bandage around the instep and bring the ends up each side of the ankle.
- Cross the ends on top and pass them around the ankle and splint.
- Cross the ends under the splint, return to the top of the ankle, cross and carry down each side of the ankle and tie under the instep.

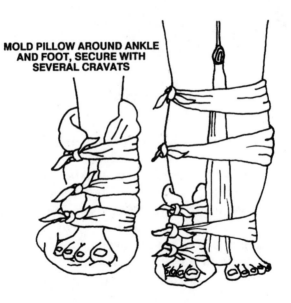

MOLD PILLOW AROUND ANKLE AND FOOT, SECURE WITH SEVERAL CRAVATS

Figures 25-26 Ankle or Foot Splint

To make an improvised splint for the ankle or foot, proceed as follows:

- Carefully fold a blanket or pillow around the ankle and foot.
- Tie the first bandage around the leg above the ankle.
- Tie the second bandage around the ankle.
- Tie the third bandage below the ankle (Figures 25-26).
- Place padding between the ankles and extend the padding above the knees (Figures 25-26).
- Place the fourth bandage around knees and tie.
- Place the fifth bandage below knees and tie.
- Place the sixth bandage around ankles and tie.

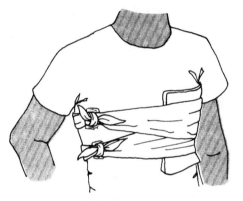

Figure 27 Rib Splint

Fracture of a rib usually is caused by a direct blow or a severe squeeze. A fracture can occur at any point along the rib. The symptoms of a fractured rib are as follows:

- Severe pain on breathing
- Tenderness over the fracture
- Deformity
- Inability to take a deep breath

Cravat bandages will immobilize fractured ribs. Place the bandages in the following order:

- Apply padding over injured ribs.
- Apply two medium cravat bandages around the chest firmly enough to afford support, centering the cravats on other side of the pain.
- Upon exhalation, tie the knots over a pad on the opposite side of the body (Figure 27). (If the cravat bandages cause more pain. loosen them.)
- Support the arm on the injured side in a sling.
- Treat for a shock as it is usually severe.
- Secure medical treatment.

KITCHEN REMEDIES

Aloe Vera–Cut a small piece of this soothing, natural infection fighter and apply directly to the wound several times daily, or slice the piece lengthwise and bandage or tape it to the area. You can use a fresh slice 1-2 times per day or overnight as needed. If you have plenty of aloe vera plants you can make inexpensive aloe juice by dropping a large amount, like cut celery, of the plant into your blender with blades covered with water, processing on high speed for a few seconds. Use the amount needed, then refrigerate the remainder in a container with a tight lid. Keeps for several days. Add less water or glycerin for a paste.

Apple Cider Vinegar–Contains silica which speeds up the rebuilding process of the bone. If you add calcium sulfate to apple cider vinegar this will also accelerate the healing process at the right time. Start slowly if you are not use to taking apple cider vinegar. Begin with 1/2 teaspoon in a cup of warm water or juice 3-4 times daily and move up to 1 teaspoon 3-4 times daily. You can use this as a nutritional support on regular bases by taking 1 teaspoon 1-2 times day building up to 1-2 tablespoons to 1-2 ounces straight or in a little juice.

Cayenne–This is good for shock and speeds healing because it stimulates blood flow. It's also an antiseptic. Sprinkle powder directly on the fracture or around it. If you are not use to cayenne, mix 1/4 to 1/2 teaspoon in a cup of warm water, then apply. You can also drink this mixture as a tea, 1-3 cups daily.

Sage–Take as a tea to help the bones rebuild and knit together 2-3 times daily or use as a poultice over the bruised or twisted bone.

Legumes (Peas and Beans)–These are called lime plants and eating them aids in building bones, ligaments, and teeth.

SINGLE HERBAL REMEDIES

Horsetail Grass–High in silica aids in rebuilding bones. Make a tea.

Oat Straw–Rich body building material for a pain compress which is high in silicon, calcium, and phosphorus. Make a fomentation or drink as tea.

Queen of the Meadow–This is great for all joint problems and it is high in vitamin A and D. Make a tea.

White Willow Bark–This is nature's aspirin that relieves pain. Use as a fomentation or make a tea.

OTHER NATURAL TREATMENTS

Sun Light–Start slowly for a few minutes 1-2 times each day and increase 5-15 minutes daily. The best time to sun is before 11 A.M. and after 4 P.M. This helps the body to produce vitamin D through the skin and aids the absorption of calcium to rebuild the bones.

Lime Water (Calcium Carbonate)–This not only rebuilds the bones, but also increases the hardness of bones and aids calcium absorption. Take 1 teaspoon 2-3 times daily in juice for about 2-3 weeks. If doing well reduce to 1/2 teaspoon 2-4 times daily.

COMMERCIALLY PREPARED HERBAL REMEDIES

Herbs: BF&C capsules and ointment (Rebuilds bones, flesh and cartilage); Fem-Mend (Balances the female hormones. (Nature's Way); Cal-Silica (natural calcium); Bone All; Calcium Citrate (calcium for tissues and nerves) (Twin Lab); Rescue Remedy (for shock and trauma) (Bach); or, liquid trace mineral (Speeds up healing for the bones and nervous system. Take 1-2 ounces 2-3 times daily in water or juice. Also, moisten a cloth or cotton with the liquid and apply to the area several times daily).

Homeopathic: Injuries; Neuralgic Pains; Emotions; or, Pain (Natra-Bio); or, Calcium Carbonate 3-6x potency. Take 2 tablets 2-3 times daily with calcium (Aids calcium absorption.).

BRUISES

Bruises occur when we bump into things, fall down, receive a blow from an object or from being pinched. These incidents cause small vessels to break under the skin without actually breaking through to the surface. A black eye would be an example. The assaulted area swells and reddens, may feel sore or painful and eventually turns a black and/or blue color.

ACTION

First, check for broken bones from the accident. Our natural instinct is to grab the injured area, which is fine, but do not let go until pain stops. Usually if you do this there is no lymphic swelling or pain.

While at a parade a young lady stepped into a hole twisting her ankle. She gave permission for me to hold the area that was hurt. After five minutes of pressure she said the pain had totally gone. She could walk without pain and enjoyed the rest of the parade.

Then wash the bruised area with a natural soap and water, and apply a natural disinfectant. You can also apply an ice pack or a cold object if needed if you were unable to hold the injured area immediately.

KITCHEN REMEDIES

Aloe Vera–Cut a small piece of this soothing, infection-fighting plant and apply directly to the bruise several times daily, or slice the piece lengthwise and bandage or tape it to the area. You can use a fresh slice 1-2 times per day or overnight as needed. If you have plenty of aloe vera plants you can make inexpensive aloe juice by dropping a large amount, like cut celery, of the plant into your blender with blades covered with water, processing on high speed for a few seconds. Take the amount needed, then refrigerate the remainder in a container with a tight lid. This keeps for several days. Add less water or glycerin for a paste to be applied to the bruise.

Witch Hazel–Responds to most injures and inflammation. Use as a fomentation.

Castor, Olive, Wheat Germ, or Safflower Oil–Any one of these oils are great in healing bruises as they soothe the soreness. Apply by spreading either a single oil or mix them together over bruised area several times a day. You also take 1/2 teaspoon 2-3 times a day with juice as an internal support.

Corn Starch–Mix corn starch with a little warm water or vegetable oil to make a paste and apply to soothe the soreness of the bruise.

Honey–Spread honey directly onto the bruise several times daily to soothe.

Potato, Carrot, or Cabbage–Use singularly or in combination to make a poultice to soothe the bruised tissues and help them heal faster.

SINGLE HERBAL REMEDIES

Echinacea–Works as an infection fighter and cleanser. Make a tea or foment the bruise.

Marigold–A great healer and anti-inflammatory for bruises. Make a tea and use as a fomentation.

St. John's Wort–This is great relief for pain, especially for nerves and the skin. Make a tea.

Bayberry–This herb encourages blood circulation thus treats bruises in a broader sense. Good for slow healing wounds. Make a tea.

COMMERCIALLY PREPARED HERBAL REMEDIES

Herbs: BF&C (Rebuilds bone, flesh and cartilage.); Comfrey or Chickweed ointment (Good healing agents and infection fighters.); Cal-Silica (natural calcium); Ex-Stress Formula (Builds nervous system.); Myrrh-Golden Seal Plus Formula (infection fighter and aids ulcerations); Rescue Remedy (for shock and trauma) (Bach); or, liquid trace minerals (Take 1-2 ounces in water or juice as needed daily. Also moisten a cloth or cotton and apply to the area several times daily as needed.).

Homeopathic: Injuries; Pain; or, Emotional (Natra-Bio); or, Injury & Backache (Medicine from Nature).

BURNS

Burns are a major cause of accidental death in the United States every year. These injuries occur from heat (liquid, steam, or fire), chemicals, or radiation. The severity, depth, and size of burns varies widely. Causes range from baths that are too hot to cigarette burns to being trapped in a burning house.

Burns are classified according to how deep and severe it is. You can't always tell how serious a burn is right away. **First degree** or minor burns are red with pain and slight swelling (see Figures 28-30). These are caused by sitting in the sun too long, touching a hot object or being scalded by steam or water.

A major or **second degree** burn (see Figures 28-30) is when the skin is broken and covers at least 10 percent of the total skin area. Blisters may form and the skin will also have a shiny appearance because of the exposed tissue and the loss of plasma. Second degree burns are often more painful than third degree burns because in the latter nerve endings are damaged. Flash burns from gasoline, direct contact with hot liquids or a serious sunburn cause these burns.

Third degree burns (see Figures 28-30) are critical and cover large areas such as the upper extremities. The skin is destroyed, muscle tissues and the bone underneath may be damaged and there is an insensitivity due to the destruction of nerve endings. The area may be charred, white, or grayish in color. Bad burns are more inclined to infection. **DO NOT PUT ANYTHING ON A THIRD DEGREE BURN.**

Chemical burns may be a result of caustic soda, household cleaning products, lime, cement, or alkalis or acids from storage batteries splattering on the body.

WARNING: In all severe burn cases, especially for third degree cases, immediately call for medical help. Do not apply any topical remedies to a third degree burn, however, you can give the victim remedies by mouth if they are conscious until medical help arrives.

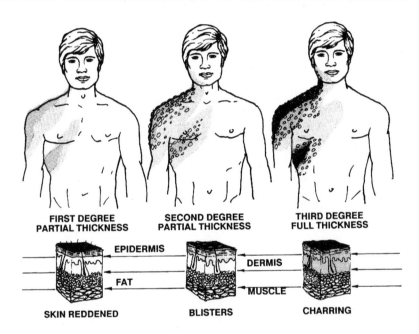

FIRST DEGREE   SECOND DEGREE   THIRD DEGREE
PARTIAL THICKNESS PARTIAL THICKNESS FULL THICKNESS

EPIDERMIS

DERMIS

FAT

MUSCLE

SKIN REDDENED   BLISTERS   CHARRING

Figures 28-30 Different Degrees of Burns

ACTION

General burns of the first degree type can be treated by immediately holding the area until pain stops which is generally in a few minutes. You can also use cold water or ice. Second degree burns require a more intense healing herb or homeopathic. If fabric is stuck to a burn, cut the cloth around the area, but not pull the fabric off that adheres to the skin. Sometimes the cloth will come off after washing and disinfecting. Do not open the blisters, or use greases or butter, and avoid dressings that are not sterile and do not wrap them tightly or the burned area may swell. Remember to never permit burned surfaces to be in contact with each other, such as areas between the fingers or toes, the ears and the side of the head, or other similar places. And, when using any of the listed remedies directly on the burned skin, be sure to warm them up a little. DO NOT PUT ANYTHING ON A THIRD DEGREE BURN.

Before using the disinfectant and suggested aid, gently wash burned area with a natural soap and water. Then apply a natural disinfectant.

Liquid Trace Mineral is one of the simplest, quickest remedies to apply. It pulls out the fiery effect, disinfects, reduces infection, causes the least searing and aids healing of the burn from the inside out. You can apply directly by spraying the burn with an atomizer, so that you do not aggravate the burned skin. You can moisten a clean cloth or cotton and lay it on the burn, keeping the covering moist. Do not remove it until the skin no longer sticks to the cloth as pulling the cloth off prematurely will open the skin. Then replace cloth still keeping the fresh cloth moist until the burn is healed.

Burns over a large area cause a loss of body fluids and electrolytes that need to be replaced. Drink 1-2 ounces of liquid trace mineral with other liquids throughout the day while recovering.

Chemical Burns–Use echinacea with equal parts of chaparral. Mix 10-20 drops or 2 capsules each 3-4 times daily and foment area. Also, you can use chlorophyll, wheat grass, or Red Clover Combination. Take 20-30 drops of one of these or use in combination, or 2 capsules each 3-4 times daily and apply as a fomentation. If the burn is tender to touch, apply one of the remedies by spraying liquid using a spray bottle.

Please Take Note: If area is bandaged do not peel the bandage all the way down to the skin or you will peel the new skin off, delaying healing and causing a secondary infection. Instead peel down to where the bandage sticks just above the skin. Then apply remedy right over the bandage. It will soak through to the skin and heal with out doing damage. Rewrap bandage or cut old bandage off, apply ointment, and wrap a few fresh bandages over the old one until the skin is healed and repeat as needed daily. Place plastic (like a bread wrapper or other types of plastic) around the bandaged area when bathing to keep it dry.

KITCHEN REMEDIES

Aloe Vera–Acts as a natural antibiotic, soothes the burned skin by drawing out the heat and aids in healing. Cut a piece of the plant and apply directly to the burn several times daily, or slice the piece lengthwise and bandage or tape it to the area if its a small burn. You can use a fresh slice 1-2 times per day or overnight as needed. If you have plenty of aloe vera plants you can make inexpensive aloe juice by dropping a large amount, like cut celery, of the plant into your blender with blades covered with water and processing on high speed for a few seconds. Use the amount needed, then refrigerate remainder in a container with a tight lid. This keeps for several days. Be sure to warm the aloe vera up before applying it to the burn. You can put the liquid in a spray bottle to spritz the warm liquid onto the burn for less painful application than spreading. Add less water or glycerin for more of a paste.

Witch Hazel–Take 1 teaspoon 3 times daily in juice and apply to the burned area.

Cayenne–Make enough paste to cover the burn by mixing olive oil with the powder. Cayenne is a natural antiseptic that speeds the healing. For a minor burn use 1/2-1 teaspoon of cayenne.

Wheat Germ Oil–Take 1 teaspoon 3-4 times daily with juice and apply by lightly spreading onto burned area to soothe the skin and fight infection.

Honey and/or Olive Oil–Take 1/2 teaspoon 2-3 times a day and apply by lightly spreading over the burned area. You may use the honey or olive oil separately or in combination to soothe skin and fight infection.

Apple Cider Vinegar–Gently apply or spray the burn with this soothing infection fighter and take 1/2 teaspoon of apple cider vinegar in juice or hot tea.

Potato or Onions–Use either one or in combination as a poultice to draw out the heat and fight infection.

SINGLE HERBAL REMEDIES

Marigold–Good for all types of burns as it speeds healing and combats inflammation. Make a tea or use as a fomentation.

St. John's Wort–This is works as an anti-inflammatory, pain reliever and heals the damaged nerve endings. Make a tea and apply as a fomentation.

OTHER NATURAL TREATMENTS

Vitamin E (200-400 IU)–Take one capsule daily and apply to the burn as it will speed healing.

> **WARNING:**   Avoid vitamin E supplementation if you are taking blood thinning medication or if you have liver disease. Don't take more than 400 I.U.s of vitamin E for any length of time unless under the guidance of a physician.

COMMERCIALLY PREPARED HERBAL REMEDIES

Herbs: For first and second degree burns, apply right away and often BF&C or Comfrey ointments for external use and take the capsules or make a tea; or, Silent Night (Aids rest and sleep.) (Nature's Way). For third degree burns use Mullein ointment. Also use Rescue Remedy for shock and trauma (Bach). Liquid trace mineral speeds healing if the burn is packed or soaked in it right away for 10-20 minutes, then every 1-2 hours. Also add 1-2 ounces of the mineral in apple juice 3-5 times daily until better and gradually reduce the amount.

Homeopathic: Injuries; or, Pain (Natra-Bio); Insomnia; Migraine Headache (Medicine from Nature); Calms (Hylands). For second to third degree burns it is best to use Cantharis 30-200X. Take 2 tablets and spray area every 30 minutes every 1-2 hours. Also dissolve 6-8 tablets in 1 quart of spring water in a spray container, shake to dissolve the tablets. Also, shake and warm up the mix before each spraying of the burned area. If using liquid trace mineral add about 20-30 drops of 30-200X potency of cantharis in 1 quart of warm spring water in a spray bottle, applying to the burns every 30 minutes to every 1-2 hours. I used this remedy and technique on a third degree explosion burn and healed the infected area in about 5-7 days with no scarring. You can also follow up with hypericum and calendula ointment and tablets for painful burns as it prevents scaring and reduces nerve pain. This is especially good for preventing muscle and nerve damage (Boericke & Tafel).

Take that amount a little longer before you begin the next level of reduction.

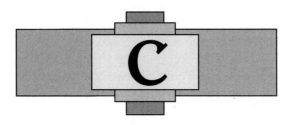

CHICKEN POX OR SHINGLES

The varicella-zoster virus causes both chicken pox and herpes zoster, also known as shingles. Chicken pox, the acute version of this disease, is typically harmless in children. Adults are also prone to this condition, although, it is harder on them. Chicken pox can be severe and even fatal in people who are taking corticosteroids or have leukemia. Chicken pox begins with a mild fever and headache, and malaise. A day or two later an itchy rash or eruption of transparent vesicles or blisters in groupings appears on different areas of the body. Rarely do chicken pox vesicles leave scars. This disease lasts about one week.

Your body is more susceptible to chicken pox when your immunity is low. Dietary habits, such as eating too many sweets, can contribute to low resistance. You want to allow the pox to break out, so do not suppress with medication or ointments, other than what I have outlined below.

Shingles, the latent phase of this viral condition, can occur at any age but usually happens after 50. Parts of the central nervous system are infected by the varicella virus causing vesicles (like in chicken pox) and pain on the skin that traces the paths taken by our sensory nerves on one side of the body, for example along the belt line. Before these eruptions occur, you may experience a fever and chills, stomach upset and a general ill feeling for three or four days. In the next day or two, vesicles appear on a red base. They can be very painful and itchy.

ACTION

Cleanse the body using enemas to flush poisons out of bowels and kidneys. Drink lots of fluids—water, natural juices, vegetable broths, soups, and natural lemonade with honey, no sugar. Warm to hot baths brings the pox to the surface as well as using warm catnip as both an enema and tea. Other helpful herbal teas are: peppermint, pleurisy root, yarrow and, especially, red raspberry. You may use a fomentation to relieve itching and help the healing process. Peppermint tea with apple cider vinegar and water relives mild itching. For severe itching use burdock and goldenseal tea. If either of these conditions get worse, you may want to consult with your doctor.

KITCHEN REMEDIES

Aloe Vera Plant–Use this remedy to stop itching and to help speed healing. Cut a several pieces of the plant and apply directly to the pox several times daily. You can use a fresh slices 1-2 times per day or overnight as needed. If you have plenty of aloe vera plants you can make inexpensive aloe paste by dropping a large amount of the plant into your blender with a little water, mixing on high speed for a few seconds. Make the amount needed, then store cold in a container with a tight lid which will keep for several days. You can also purchase aloe vera gel from the health food store.

Apple Cider Vinegar–Dilute this infection fighter with a little water and apply directly to rash with a clean hand, cotton cloth, or spray on as needed.

Sage–Drink a cup 1-3 times daily to fight the infection and to soothe the pox. Also, paint or spray the poxed area with the tea as needed.

Witch Hazel–Paint area with straight witch hazel or dilute a little with water and apply with a clean hand, cotton cloth, or spray on. This astringent speeds the healing of the pox sores.

Celery–Make a juice from fresh celery in a blender or juicer, then drink 2-4 ounces straight or mixed with other juices. Take as often as needed. Celery juice calms the nervous system. You may also paint the pox area if you are not allergic to celery.

SINGLE HERBAL REMEDIES

Any of the following herbal remedies may be used as a fomentation and be taken internally. For fomenting apply the warm liquid or oil with a cloth or directly onto the pox area.

Red Raspberry–An effective astringent which is great for all types of viral eruptive problems, like chicken pox and measles. Use as a tea or fomentation.

Tansy–This is a great pain reliever for eruptive skin diseases. Give tea in small, repeated doses because extra large doses may cause abdominal cramps. Do not use for extended periods. You can mix tansy with other herbs and foment the area or soak in bath.

> **WARNING:**   Do not use tansy while pregnant.

OTHER NATURAL TREATMENTS

Soak Bath–You can mix 1/2 cup of apple cider vinegar in bath water and soak about 20-30 minutes. Also, you may do the same with 1-2 cups of baking soda in the bath water or dilute 1 teaspoon in cup of hot water and apply with a hand or cotton cloth as needed.

Hot baths bring out the pox because the heat expands the skin and inner body tissue drawing the toxins to the skins surface and into the water. While filling the tub with hot water suited to your body add single or combination of herbs desired. As alternatives you can use 1-2 cups of epsom salts or 1 cup of aloe vera. Soaking is also great for relaxing the entire body for sleep.

COMMERCIALLY PREPARED REMEDIES

Herbs: IF Formula (for inflammation and infections); Ex-Stress Formula (Calms the nervous system.); AKN (A good skin support.); Kalmin (An antispasmodic extract that relaxes the nervous system.); Cal-Silica Formula (Natural calcium that supports nerves and tissues.); Liveron (Cleanses the liver.); Silent Night Formula (A sleep aid.); BF&C, Chickweed and Comfrey ointment (A great healer of various skin sores.) (Nature's Way); or, liquid trace minerals (Apply to sores with cotton, use 1-2 cups in a for adults, 1/2 cup for older children and 1/4 cup for younger children and babies. Also take 1/2 ounce 1-2 times daily in water or juice to heal from the inside-out.)

Homeopathic: Neuralgic Pain; Pain; Calendala, Hypericum, or Detoxification (Natra-Bio). See a homeopath for additional help.

CHOKING

Choking can occur when any kind of obstruction in the air passage results in unconsciousness and respiratory arrest. A variety of foods cause choking, but meat is the most common because people do not chew the meat enough to break the piece down. When the airway is completely obstructed the person is unable to speak, breathe, or cough and will clutch the neck which is the universal distress signal for choking. If the choking person is not helped, unconsciousness from lack of oxygen will result and death will follow quickly if prompt action is not taken.

ACTION

There are several ways to relieve the situation using an abdominal thrust, the first is the Heimlich Maneuver (see Figure 31). Second, if you are by yourself you can still use an abdominal thrust by using a chair (see Figure 32). And thirdly, if the person is laying down (see Figure 33).

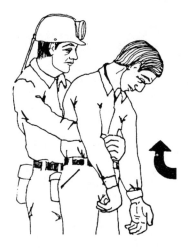

Figure 31 Heimlich Maneuver

- Determine if airway obstruction is partial or complete.
- If partial obstruction (air exchange), encourage victim to cough.
- If there is no air exchange, stand behind the victim and place your arms around the victim's waist.
- Grasp one fist in your other hand and position the thumb side of your fist against the middle of the victim's abdomen just above the navel and well below rib cage.
- Do not squeeze victim.
- Press your fist into the victim's abdominal area with a quick upward thrust.
- Repeat the procedure if necessary.

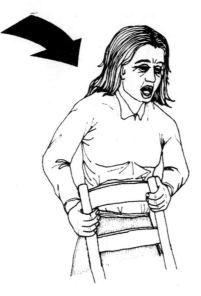

Figure 32 Abdominal Thrust Using a Chair

The victim of an obstructed airway, who is alone may use his/her own fist, as described previously, or bend over the back of a chair and exert downward pressure.

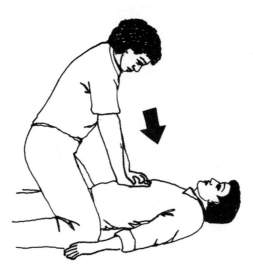

Figure 33 Abdominal Thrust Laying Down

- Position victim on his/her back, face up.
- Straddle victim's hips, if possible.
- Place the heel of one hand against the middle of the victim's abdomen between the rib cage and the navel with fingers pointing toward the victim's chest.
- Place your other hand on top of the first.
- Move your shoulders directly over the victim's abdomen.
- Press into the victim's abdominal area with a quick upward thrust.
- Do 6 to 10 thrusts.
- Attempt artificial ventilation
- Repeat the procedures until obstruction is cleared.

COLDS AND FLU

The common cold has eluded modern medical treatment. However, there are many natural remedies that can prevent and even cure this ailment. A cold is actually an upper respiratory infection caused by a number of different viruses. Symptoms run the gamut from a runny nose or eyes, sneezing, coughing, sneezing as well as sinus and chest congestion. There is usually no fever associated with a cold, although small children and infants may experience a mild rise in body temperature. Most colds last four to 10 days. They aren't serious unless a secondary bacterial infection develops, for example in the ear or sinuses.

Unlike a cold, the flu is characterized by a fever and chills. Aches and pains, typically in the back and legs, are also part and parcel of influenza. This viral condition also includes coughing, headache, sensitivity to light, aching eyeballs and the other respiratory symptoms that accompany a cold. Complications due to the flu, such as pneumonia, are more serious than with colds. This is particularly true of the very young and very old.

WARNING: If your home remedies are not helping an elderly patient, a baby, or small child with the flu, seek professional medical help. Always call your doctor if your infant has a fever.

ACTION

The most important actions are to keep yourself warm and rest. Drink plenty of water and vegetable broth or juice to avoid dehydration and constipation. If you must drink fruit juices, dilute them half and half with water. Bathe frequently and change your bedding often. For patients with a fever, See "Fever." Use any of the recommended remedies.

KITCHEN REMEDIES

Cinnamon, Ginger, or Sage–Use either fresh or powdered as a tea and in a hot soak bath. Put 1/4 teaspoon of cinnamon or ginger powder in a cup of hot water or in the juice of 1/2 of a lemon, warmed up, with a little honey for taste. Drink it down. You may add 1 teaspoon of sage to the ginger and cinnamon tea if you wish. For a hot soak bath, use 1 teaspoon of cinnamon, ginger, or 1 tablespoon of sage (see below).

Sage–This works as a natural antibacterial and is good for nausea. Drink as a tea by itself or with other herbs.

Ginger–Use this if you have a sore throat, headache, bronchial congestion, or stuffy nose. Chop or juice about a 1/2 teaspoon of fresh ginger or use 1/4 teaspoon of the juice and mix it with a cup of hot tea or juice. Drink several times a day.

Garlic–This pungent bulb has been dubbed Russian penicillin. Use fresh garlic that is grated, squeezed, and soaked in apple cider vinegar. Take 1 teaspoon straight or in juice or tea every 1-2 hours. Garlic helps to clear the cold and warms the body. You may add 1/4 teaspoon of cinnamon or cayenne to the tea.

Garlic and Onion–Chop or juice about 1/2 teaspoon each of fresh garlic and onion, or, use 1/4 teaspoon of juice, mix the vegetables in a cup of hot tea or juice, and drink several times a day to clear out the toxins. Teas to use are sage, cinnamon, or catnip and you may add a natural sweetener such as honey. You can also use garlic oil from the health food store.

Apple Cider Vinegar–Cleanses the body's system. Mix 1/4 tablespoon to a cup of hot water. You may add a 1/4 teaspoon of cinnamon, 1/4 teaspoon of sage and drink several times throughout the day. Honey can be used to sweeten.

Horseradish–Freshly grated, chopped, or diced horseradish is mixed in with a little apple cider vinegar. Begin with a little and gradually increase it a little each time by mixing it in food at each meal until you can tolerate at least 1/4 teaspoon or more. Other warm or hot peppers can also be added in food. You can mix a little in a juice 1-2 times daily or, hold a little in the mouth to open up the sinuses, kill the germs, and gargling if you have a sore throat then spit out.

Lemon–Fresh is best to work as an antiseptic. Squeeze the juice of a 1/2 of a lemon in a cup of hot water, natural sweetener such as honey is optional. You can also add ginger, sage, mint tea, or a little cayenne and if the taste is too strong use some more lemon to dilute the mixture.

Cloves–Promotes sweating and breaks up the congestion. Use whole cloves if possible. Steep 1 teaspoon in a cup of hot water or small sauce pan for few minutes. Strain and drink a 1/2 cup several times daily as needed.

SINGLE HERBAL REMEDIES

Echinacea–Fights all infections and builds the immune system. Make a tea. For upset stomachs, flu and diarrhea, you may add catnip to the tea.

Elder Flower–For severe colds or congestion mix a 1/2 teaspoon of peppermint and 1 teaspoon of elder flower and steep 5 minutes. Or use 1 capsule of each in 1 pint of hot water steeping 3 minutes. Drink 4-6 ounces ever 1-2 hours. Elder flower is great for all forms of colds and fevers, even for children and babies, and it never fails.

Pleurisy Root–For stronger infections, particularly if the congestion moves to or threatens to move into the lungs, use this remedy. An excellent sweating agent, especially for the flu, fevers, pneumonia, or other lung problems. To overcome chills, you can also add a little cayenne to the pleurisy root. Make a tea.

Eucalyptus Oil–Inhale this decongestant oil. Put 4-6 drops in hot water then with a towel draped over the head and bowl, breathe in. Do this as needed to clear sinuses. If you have a humidifier, put a few drops to ease breathing.

Red Raspberry–Particularly good if diarrhea is part of your flu. Make a tea.

Spearmint/Peppermint–Helps to calm an upset stomach. Use separately, or in combination with other herbs, for nausea and vomiting. It's ability to induce sweating makes it valuable for treating fevers. You can inhale peppermint (see Eucalyptus) for a stuffed-up nose. Additionally, you may combine either with pleurisy root for pneumonia. Make a tea with either mint.

White Willow Bark–A natural aspirin that helps with lightly aching bones and chills. This was used by the Native Americans. Make a tea. (See "Fevers" for information on when to treat a fever and chills.)

OTHER NATURAL TREATMENTS

Soak Bath–A great relaxing tonic for the whole body and improves circulation. The heat expands pores in the skin drawing congestion out of the body. While filling the tub with hot water suited to your body add the cinnamon, ginger, sage, or 1-2 cups of epsom salt.

Vitamin B-6–Good for light to heavy bone aches and chills. Take 1 (50 mg) tablet or capsule per hour while body aches, up to 6 hours.

> **WARNING:** It is important that the vitamins be a natural brand, such as Kal, Twin Lab, or Schiff. High doses for a long period of time may cause peripheral neuropathy, or numbness and tingling in your hands and feet.

If this does not help aches or chills, then take boneset tea or homeopathic boneset 200X (usually this can be acquired from a homeopath).

COMMERCIALLY PREPARED HERBAL REMEDIES

Herbs: Fenu-Thyme Formula (for congestive mucus); Herbal Influence Formula; GL Formula (Cleanses and supports the glands.); Breath-Aid (respiratory support); HAS Original Formula (Use this if you are sensitive to Pseudoephedrine for nasal congestion) or HAS Fast-Acting Formula (Contains Pseudoephedrine.); Comfrey-Mullein-Garlic Syrup (for coughs); Immunaid; Winter Care Formula; Echinacea Combination (May take either hot or cold, but hot is the best.); Naturalax 1, 2, or 3 or Aloe Lax (Either relieves sluggish, toxic bowels.) (Nature's Way); Boneset (Great for severe flu problems, deep chills, aching, and fevers used by Native Americans. Take 1/2 teaspoon of extract or open 1 capsule in 1/2 cup of hot water stir and steep with saucer on top about 5 minutes. Drink one every hour until the patient sweats it out and symptoms leave. You can also swallow 2 capsules with a fluid 2-4 times a day.)

Homeopathic: Depending on the symptoms use, Cold; Cough; Flu; Fever; Sore Throat; Exhaustion; or, Laxative (Natra-Bio); Bone-set 30-200X (Works great for deep chills and aches.); Cold & Flu; Earache; Fatigue; Sinusitis; or, Teething (Medicine from Nature).

COLIC

Colic is a spasmodic pain usually identified with babies. In infants, this symptom is accompanied by irritability and crying. The name colic, which means of the colon, implies this condition is due to intestinal upset. However, we are puzzled as to why infants up to four months of age are afflicted. Theories range from an immature nervous system, overfeeding, air swallowing, and emotional upset. Food allergies or sensitivity may also be a factor. Regardless of the cause, babies seem to outgrow this. However, that is little consolation for parents who must deal with a crying and hurting infant.

WARNING: Do not give anyone laxatives who has acute abdominal pain as this may be a case of appendicitis.

ACTION

Colic in adults may be due to a variety of causes. In this book, I'm going to concentrate on digestive problems and remedies. A simple place to start is to improve your diet by decreasing sugars, fats, salt, caffeine, and alcohol. Try better food combining or abstain from suspected allergic foods. Common allergic foods include wheat, dairy products (milk, cheese, butter, ice cream), soy, corn, eggs, citrus fruits (oranges, grapefruits, lemons, limes), tomatoes, chocolate, and sugar. Watch food labels closely for these foods. Soy, corn, and sugar are common food additives. (See "Allergies.")

You may fast with water or juices for a few days (please review instruction for fasting under "How to use this book"). If you plan to do this for more than three days, visit with a professional trained in therapeutic fasting. Drink at least six glasses of water each day to keep the bowels functioning properly. Another alternative is to take digestive enzymes one half hour before each meal.

If your baby is colicky and you are not breast feeding, change from a cow milk-based formula to a soy-based formula. If you are nursing and are occasionally supplementing your baby with formula, try using goat's milk, soy, or another nut milk. Avoid cow's milk before a baby is six months old as this milk can induce food allergies. If you are nursing exclusively, check your own diet for possible food allergies. Also try eliminating caffeine, alcohol, garlic and onions, and gassy vegetables such as broccoli and cabbage. Give the remedy to a baby in a bottle.

If there are repeated colic attacks, then check with your doctor.

KITCHEN REMEDIES

Baking Soda–Mix a 1/4 teaspoon of this natural antacid with 4 ounces of warm water and, if desired, add some honey to sweeten. For *older children* (5-12 years old) give 3-4 ounces. Have the child sit upright and sip the mixture slowly over a period of about 30 minutes, allowing them to belch freely. *Adults* need to drink the entire 4 ounces in the same manner as the older child.

WARNING: Unless your doctor supervises you, do not give baking soda to children under 5 years old. Don't use more than 1/2 teaspoon 8 times per day if under 60, or 4 times a day if over 60. Don't use this maximum amount for more than two weeks. Don't use baking soda if you're on a sodium restricted diet.

Sage–Soothes and settles the intestinal system and works as an antiseptic. This is a great relief for colic. Make a tea.

Lemon–Squeeze 1/2-1 fresh lemon into a cup of warm water. Honey can be added for sweetening. For *adults* and *older children* sip lemon juice slowly, sitting upright. Administer 1 ounce of the lemon juice in a baby bottle for *infants*.

WARNING: Do not give honey to babies under one year of age.

Castor Oil–Rub across abdomen to soothe. You can apply heat with a towel wrapped around a heating pad.

Olive Oil–This is a wonderful old German nurse remedy to settle the stomach and release intestinal gas. For *adults:* Take 1/2-1 teaspoon first thing in the morning on an empty stomach, then don't eat for 1 hour. For *children* or *babies*: put a few drops in water or juice depending on the age.

Apple Cider Vinegar–Mix 1 teaspoon per quart of warm water to break up the gas in the stomach and intestinal tract. Drink 1-3 ounces according to the age of the individual and repeat as needed.

Ginger–Great for lower stomach problems as it soothes and settles. Ginger tea can be used in an enema as well as a drink.

SINGLE HERBAL REMEDIES

Remember that the dosages listed below are for *adults*. Check the Dosage Information at the front of the book to adjust for infants and children.

Peppermint–This soothes and settles the system. Make a tea. The tea can also be used in enema (see below).

Catnip–Soothes and settles nerves and gas problems. You can add a few drops of garlic to the tea. Also catnip tea can be used as enema (see below).

Fennel–Good for problems with gas and bowels, and aids liver and gallbladder. Use the tea as an enema or drink it.

> **WARNING:** Large amounts of fennel can disturb the nervous system.

Chamomile and/or Mint Teas–Both of these teas soothes and settles the nervous system. You may add a few drops of garlic oil to mint tea.

Wild Yam–Relieves gas, soothes and settles the intestinal system. Make a tea.

Valerian Root–Take 1/2-1 teaspoon of straight valerian root or 1 capsule as needed. This works as a sedative and nerve tonic.

OTHER NATURAL TREATMENTS

Enema–This technique relieves bowel gas and releases the toxic fecal matter. For *adults:* Mix 1 teaspoon of apple cider vinegar per quart of water in a bag of warm distilled or spring water.

For *babies* or *children:* Mix 10-15 drops of apple cider vinegar to warm water, fill a Fleet baby enema bottle. You can get this bottle at a drug store which will be filled with a chemical enema that needs to be poured out and replaced with the natural enema.

COMMERCIALLY PREPARED HERBAL REMEDIES

Herbs: Kalmin (Anti-Spasmodic Extract); KOL-X (for gas); Ex-Stress Extract (Calms nervous system.); Cal-Silica Formula (Supports nervous system.) (Nature's Way); or, Liquid Calcium for children.

Homeopathic: Laxative; Teething; or, Candida Yeast (Can cause gas and bloatiness.) (Natra-Bio); Calms (Calms nervous system.); Colic: or, Teething (Hylands); or, Indigestion & Gas; Teething; or, Colic (Medicine from Nature).

CONSTIPATION

Constipation is usually due to a poor diet that is lacking in fiber, improper food combinations, a lack of the proper amount of daily intake of water, exercise, and avoiding the "call" or "urge." One bowel movement daily is not sufficient. If you eat 3 meals daily times 7 days a week you consume 21 meals. If you only have 1 bowel movement daily times 7 days is only 7 bowel movements per week. This is not even 50 percent elimination of the food you had in one week. Now multiply this by the number of weeks in one year! Get the idea!

> **WARNING:** Do not give laxatives to anyone with acute abdominal pain as this may be a case of appendicitis.

ACTION

Improve your diet with fiber and laxative foods like prunes, fruit, grains, drink more water, and exercise. If your problem becomes chronic or severe, use an enema for immediate relief and take a natural remedy for help. Do **not** take harsh laxatives that irritate the bowels nor mineral oil which blocks vitamin A absorption. Use natural foods or herbs to aid the bowels, such as, olive, wheat germ, and castor oils instead as lubricating nutrients as well as the other suggested remedies.

KITCHEN REMEDIES

Aloe Vera–With the outer bark still on the leaf, aloe vera makes a good laxative. If you grow a lot of aloe vera, you can clip off a piece, blend it in water or juice and drink daily.

Sage–Drink a cup of tea 1-3 times a day to break up the gases. Steep 1/4 teaspoon of sage in a cup of water adding a pinch of ginger and cinnamon. To sweeten, use honey.

Lemon–Every morning before breakfast, squeeze 1/2 of a lemon into a cup of hot water and drink. Then drink 4-6 ounces more every hour, stopping at 6 P.M. to allow the bladder to empty before bedtime. This procedure lubricates the bowels and assists to increase bowel movements. Additionally, eat more fiber.

Figs–Eat fresh figs when possible as they are a natural laxative.

WARNING:　Eat only a few if you have any blood sugar problems as figs are very high in natural sugar.

Prunes–Best to use prunes after they have been soaked overnight in mineral water or apple juice. In addition, you can add hot water to the liquid the prunes are soaking in and drink it or add it to the prunes and eat them. Prune juice is fine, however, fresh prunes give more bulk helping the bowels to move and have more nutritional value.

Castor and Olive Oils–Warm either oil or mix both and rub across the abdomen. Castor oil breaks up the encrusted matter in the intestines and the olive oil is a nutrient and rebuilder of tissue. You can also lay a towel over abdomen, place a heating pad on the towel on low heat and cover with another towel for 20-30 minutes. It is good to cut the heat off before going to sleep, but, leaving the oil on overnight. Neither of these oils will stain sheets. The best therapy is three nights of castor oil and three nights of olive oil.

SINGLE HERBAL REMEDIES

Chaparral–A great cleanser and rebuilder of the bowels. Make a tea.

Dandelion–This is another great cleanser especially for the liver. Make a tea.

Senna Leaves–This is a strong action remedy for chronic problems in adults. Only use this for temporary relief. It's best to address the cause of your constipation. Blend senna with other herbs such as fennel or ginger, or dilute. Start with 10-15 drops or 1-2 capsules in a cup of hot or room temperature water and take 1-2 times daily.

Turkey Rhubarb–This works very nicely as a cleanser because it purges the bowels and then its astringent quality removes any remaining debris in the colon. Make a tea by putting 10-15 drops of the liquid extract or 1 opened capsule in a cup of hot or room tem-perature water, or in juice. Drink 1-2 times a day depending on bowel reaction and need. Best to combine with other herbs to downplay any griping that may occur. **Note:** This herb may cause your urine to turn very yellow or red.

COMMERCIALLY PREPARED HERBAL REMEDIES

Herbs: NaturaLax 2, or AloeLax (Either aids the action of the bow-els); Liveron (Cleanses the liver and gallbladder.); Ex-Stress extract or capsules (Tones and relaxes nerves.) (Nature's Way); Fletcher's Castoria (Made from fig extract and works through the liver for proper stimulation and cleansing. Especially good for children, but adults can take 2-3 times their dosage.

Homeopathic: Laxative; Detoxification; Emotional; or, Candida Yeast (Natra-Bio); Colic; Constipation & Hemorrhoids; or, Indigestion & Gas (Medicine from Nature); or, Colic; Calms; or, Diarrhea (Hylands).

CONVULSIONS

A convulsion, or seizure, begins with the person becoming uncon-scious. Depending on what part or how much of the brain is involved, convulsive symptoms may include jerking and stiffening of the body, spasms, the eyes rolling up, heavy and coarse breathing, frothing from the mouth, a change in skin color, staggering, unintelligible sounds or merely a blank expression. In extreme instances, vomiting, urination, or soiling can occur.

Epilepsy, eclampsia (a serious condition occurring during or directly after pregnancy), poisons, fever, lack of oxygen, an extreme drop in blood sugar as well as an injury from an accident may bring a convulsion on. If the person is already susceptible to seizures, then sound or light may induce convulsive activity.

> **WARNING:**   If the convulsions are continuous, from severe poisoning, the person is unconscious after the episode, or a pregnant woman has seizures, call for medical help immediately. Also check for a medical identification bracelet or necklace to see if the person is epileptic or has an allergy to a medication.

ACTION

During the seizure, lower the person to the ground in order to keep them from falling and hurting themselves, letting the convulsion run its course. Loosen clothing around the neck and place a pillow under the person's head. If possible, place a soft object, such as a folded handkerchief, between the person's teeth. Generally the convulsion will be over in a few minutes. At the end of the seizure, turn the person on their side to allow any fluids to drain from the mouth. Then keep the person calm, quiet, warm, and comfortable. Check for medical warnings on medical bracelets or in their wallet. Apply a remedy and call doctor if needed. If the convulsion is due to a known ingested poison, read label for appropriate action. If it's due to an unknown poison, call a Poison Control Center (see "Poisoning") or your local hospital. If a pregnant woman seizes, transport her immediately to the hospital. Convulsions in pregnancy are usually due to eclampsia, a life threatening ailment. Convulsions may be from a drop in blood sugar, so give a little honey or a small piece of candy if the person is conscious.

KITCHEN REMEDIES

Cayenne–If the person is unconscious, mix some powder with water or vegetable oil and rub on the feet, palms, or in navel. Cayenne helps to balance the blood and blood pressure. When the person is revived, have them drink a cup of warm or hot water with 1/4 teaspoon of cayenne in it. You can also use cayenne oil from the health food store topically or in a tea.

Honey–Can help raise blood sugar if it has dropped too low. Take a little honey or other natural sweetener and hold it in the mouth. If the person is unconscious rub a little in the navel or on the bottom of the feet. The sugar content will absorb through the skin into the blood stream and balance the low blood sugar drop. This may help bring back consciousness. If you are prone to seizures, you can also carry some hard candy or raisins in a pocket, purse, or briefcase to help keep blood sugar stable.

SINGLE HERBAL REMEDIES

Catnip, Chamomile, Passion Flower, Garlic, Valerian Root, Wild Yam–All of these act as antispasmodics as they relax the nerves and muscles. Make a tea.

Peppermint or Spearmint–Soothes and relaxes the muscles and nerves acting as antispasmodics. Make a tea.

Red Clover–Cleanses the blood and relaxes the nervous system. Make a tea.

COMMERCIALLY PREPARED HERBAL REMEDIES

Herbs: Kalmin (anti-spasmodic extract); PC Formula (Balances pancreas and blood sugar.); Ex-Stress extract or capsules (Calms nervous system.); Cal-Silica (Natural calcium for nerves) (Nature's Way); Rescue Remedy (for shock and trauma) (Bach); Calms (Hylands); Calcium Citrate (Twin Lab.) or Vegetable Calcium (Schiff).

Homeopathic: Emotional; Nervousness; Exhaustion; Raw Adrenal; or, Pancreas (Natra-Bio); Fatigue; or, Tension Headache (Medicine from Nature).

COUGHING

Coughing acts as a protective mechanism that helps clear foreign material or excess mucus from clogging the larynx and respiratory tract. Because a cough serves a purpose, it's not always desirable to suppress it. Rather, try to find out the cause of the cough and treat appropriately. However, occasionally it's necessary to temporarily suppress the cough so the patient can rest.

When and where a cough occurs can offer clues as to its cause. If other symptoms such as runny nose, sore throat, and sneezing accompany a cough, it is most probably due to a viral infection (see "Colds/Flu"). If a cough is of a long-term nature and is productive or wet and persists for months or years, is probably due to chronic bronchitis. Wheezing may be due to asthma. Asthma can be aggravated by allergens, exercise, stress, cigarette smoke or other noxious substances (see "Asthma"). You can develop a cough merely due to allergies without having asthma as well (see "Allergies"). A person who smokes and wakes each morning with a hacking cough most likely has "smoker's" cough.

Whooping cough is a very contagious, bacterial infection that includes sneezing, watery eyes, malaise, loss of appetite, and a characteristic nighttime cough that sounds like a "whoop." This condition is serious in the very young (under two years old) and the elderly.

Croup is a viral infection of both the upper and lower respiratory system. An upper respiratory infection usually precedes this condition. When croup finally develops, a barking-like cough is apparent that is most intense at night and, in young children especially, is coupled with fear.

ACTION

Usually infections are due to sluggish bowels, lack of water, and poor diet. Correct the kind and types of food you are eating, use an enema and implant to help clear out toxins, and drink a proper amount of water daily. Determine if the cause of the cough is from allergies, an infection, asthma, smoking, exposure to poisonous substances, and apply one of the suggested remedies.

KITCHEN REMEDIES

Apple Cider Vinegar–Mix 1 teaspoon of apple cider vinegar in 4-6 ounces of warm water and drink it all down at one time and cover up. You may add 1-2 tablespoons for honey to the apple cider vinegar, sipping little throughout the day for coughing.

Lemon and Honey–Besides coughing this is good for a sore throat or strained voice. Squeeze several drops of lemon in a tablespoon of honey as needed for coughing throughout the day. Also, this remedy is great as a tea by mixing the juice of 1/2 of a lemon and 1/2 teaspoon of honey in a cup of hot water and drinking a cup every hour. Add a pinch of cayenne to help speed the healing. Fresh lemons are better than the premixed lemon juice. I have found this to be one of the best remedies when no other herb is working.

Sage–Drink as a tea or use as a gargle for a sore throat. Sage works as an antiseptic and antibiotic. You may add a pinch of cayenne, cinnamon, ginger, or honey to the tea or 1/4 teaspoon of thyme to reduce mucus.

Onion and Garlic–Grate, chop, dice, or mince a fresh onion and garlic to use as natural antibiotics and antivirals. Then soak the vegetables, overnight if possible, in a quart of apple cider vinegar with 1-2 tablespoons of honey. Strain and take 1 teaspoon and allowing it to slowly trickle down the throat, coating it. You can mix the concoction in a cup of hot water and drink slowly as tea. For additional relief, first apply vegetable or olive oil over the chest and feet, then rub the mixture over this area. Cover up the chest and feet to keep warm.

Horseradish–Mix some horseradish with a little food or juice, or hold it in the mouth, a little at time, for a few minutes and then let the portion slide down throat to give relief from coughing. You can also mix the horseradish with a little honey. Take as needed. To help decongest the chest, rub a little olive or vegetable over the area, then spread some horseradish. You can also place a bowl of horseradish by the bed to assist easier breathing during the night.

SINGLE HERBAL REMEDIES

Cayenne–You can mix this with other herbs in addition to using it as a single remedy. Cayenne is a general tonic and stimulant that wards off colds, as well as being an antiseptic. Take as a tea by putting 5-10 drops of the liquid in juice or open one capsule in a cup of hot water. Drink 2-3 times per day.

Garlic Oil–You can mix garlic oil, a natural antibiotic, in with apple cider vinegar and honey if you do not want to take it straight. Make a tea. You can also hold garlic oil in the mouth, allowing it to dissolve slowly like cough syrup.

Fenugreek–Tea made from fenugreek is good for clearing mucus and congestion in the chest. Thus it helps a cough loosen this debris. Make a tea.

Elder Flower–Apply to the throat and neck area for its antiseptic and cleansing properties, especially of catarrh. Use as a fomentation and make a tea.

Pleurisy Root–Clears out congestion from the lungs and chest area, thereby aiding the respiratory system. Make a tea.

Mullein–If you have the croup, this remedy works well as a decongestant that is particularly good for lungs. It's specific for hard, sore coughs caused by bronchitis. Make a tea.

OTHER NATURAL TREATMENTS

Soak Bath–Because this is so relaxing, it will ease your cough as well. While filling the tub with hot water suited to your body add single or combination of herbs desired. Also can use 1-2 cups of epsom salts, 1 cup of aloe vera, apple cider vinegar, baking soda, or a few drops of eucalyptus oil.

COMMERCIALLY PREPARED HERBAL REMEDIES

Herbs: Original HAS Formula (This is without the Pseudoephedrine that may over-activate the heart.); Breath-Aid Formula (respiratory and congestion help); Fenu-Thyme (Thins and moves the mucus out.); Herbal Influence Formula (colds); Comfrey-Mullein-Garlic Syrup (for cough spasms); IF Formula (for coughing, inflammation and the immune system); or, GL Formula (for glands).

Homeopathic: Cough; Fever; Sinus; Sore Throat; Cold; Earache; Flu; Pain; Cold; Detoxification; or, Laxative (Natra-Bio); or, Cold & Flu; Dry Cough; Earache; or, Sinusitis (Medicine from Nature).

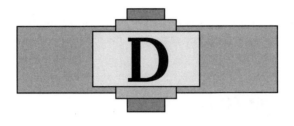

DEPRESSION

Everyone occasionally suffers from depression, the "blues," melancholy, or low spirits. In fact, depression can be viewed as a defense against frustrating situations. It allows one to withdraw from life for awhile, preserving inner resources to heal and regroup. Typical depression symptoms include change in appetite, difficulty thinking or concentrating, decreased energy, loss of libido, anxiety, lack of interest in anything, becoming withdrawn, and feelings of hopelessness or worthlessness. With time and reassurance, people generally rebound from minor bouts of depression.

Severe depression, on the other hand, is a serious problem that requires professional help. Warning signs are unrelenting depression, extreme agitation or mental sluggishness, delusions, total withdrawal from activities, severe physical symptoms (that have no other explanation), and suicidal tendencies. If a person becomes hyperactive either with or without depression, then a manic disorder is suspected.

WARNING: Professional mental health help is needed in extreme cases of depression. If a person is suicidal, seek professional psychiatric services immediately. If you or someone you're treating has or a history of addiction, be cautious in using sedative herbs.

ACTION

If this is a situational depression, try to deal with the source or cause of the problem, such as loss of job, death, divorce, or relationship break up by reassuring the person. Sometimes it is best to have someone to "talk it out" with. Other times it's best to get your mind off of the problem, so, go out to do other things, stay busy, see a funny movie, laugh, or cry. Meanwhile try one of the remedies to support the system.

KITCHEN REMEDIES

Catnip, Chamomile, Peppermint, or Sage–Brew any of these teas to relax and calm the nerves, either separately or combine them, drinking a cup of tea 2-4 times daily. If you have the loose leaves in your pantry make the tea from the directions in the front of the book, otherwise, you may find tea bags at your grocery or health store. To sweeten the tea use honey.

Honey–Take a spoonful directly into the mouth if depression is due to low sugar. This is a temporary measure.

Raisins–Eat a good handful if problem is identified as due to low sugar. This is a temporary measure.

SINGLE HERBAL REMEDIES

Red Raspberry–Calms nerves as it balances the hormones. Make a tea.

Valerian Root–Relaxes system. Make a tea.

St. John's Wort–This herb is classically used for nerve pain. But we're now finding out it's useful in cases of depression too. Make a tea.

Wormwood–A great relaxant. Make a tea.

WARNING: Habitual use may cause vomiting, convulsions and restlessness. Overdose is identified by cramps, dizziness, intoxication, and delirium.

COMMERCIALLY PREPARED REMEDIES

Herbs: Cal-Silica Formula (Natural calcium that supports the nerves.); Siberian Ginseng Root Extract (Balances the male/female system.); PC Formula (Balances blood sugar.); Silent Night (for insomnia and calms nervous system); Naturalax 1, 2, or 3 (for toxic bowels); Calcium Citrate (Twin Lab) or, Vegetable Calcium (Schiff) (Either supports nervous system.); liquid trace minerals (Balances trace minerals. Take about 1/2 ounces 2 times daily in juice.); Rescue Remedy (Take through the day as needed for nervousness, shock and trauma.).

Homeopathic: Nervousness; Menstrual; Menopause; Laxative; Exhaustion; Emotional; Candida Yeast; PMS; or, Detoxification (Natra-Bio.); or, Fatigue; Insomnia; Menopause; or, PMS (Nature's Way); See a homeopath for additional help.

DIARRHEA

Diarrhea, a symptom that can occur as part of a number of different conditions, varies depending on its cause, duration, and severity. Typically, diarrhea is recognized by increased frequency, volume, and fluidity of bowel movements. When blood, mucus, pus, or fatty substances are seen in the stools, disease may be present. Colitis, flu, reactions or allergies to food, dysentery, hepatitis, diverticulitis, cholera, bacterial toxins, parasitic infections such as Giardia, viral infections, malabsorption, eating too much fresh fruit, malnutrition, laxative abuse, emotional-mental causes are all possibilities. Bowels are usually watery, runny, gassy, and you may experience vomiting, fever, cramping, and a spastic colon. Excessive loss of fluid and electrolytes can cause great weakness and, in extreme cases, even death.

WARNING: If you suspect diarrhea is due to food poisoning or it cannot be abated by a natural remedy, call for medical help.

ACTION

Sudden diarrhea can be caused by food poisoning caused by bacterial contamination. Shellfish, especially clams and oysters, or food with spoiled mayonnaise, such as potato or chicken salad or hollandaise sauce, are common targets. If you have become ill after eating in a restaurant or at a friend's house, be sure to notify them. (see "Food Poisoning"). Also, check for other food sensitivities or allergies from wheat, milk, sugar, and other common allergy causing foods.

For chronic diarrhea, have your doctor check for candida, giardia, or salmonella infections, or Crohn's disease. Use the suggested remedy for relief orally and as a rectum implant.

KITCHEN REMEDIES

Sage–You may drink this antibiotic tea straight or add 1/2 teaspoon of cinnamon or a little peppermint. To sweeten mix in some honey.

Apple Cider Vinegar–Works as an antiseptic and helps kill or slow most of the parasites that may be causing the diarrhea. Take 1/2-1 teaspoon in 4-6 ounces of water 3-4 times daily as needed.

Allspice–Stops the diarrhea and eases stomach pain. Take 1 teaspoon of allspice simmered a few minutes in unsweetened blackberry juice or wine or if you do not have either of the liquids, then take it undiluted. Cool to taste and give 1 teaspoon to 1 ounce every 2-4 hours. Allspice can also be added to other remedies.

Cloves–Settles and cleanses the stomach. Steep 1-2 tablespoons of cloves for 15 minutes in quart of water. Strain and take 1/2 tablespoon either straight or in a cup of warm water or hot herbal tea as needed.

Carob Powder–Makes a great cleanser of the stomach and intestines and attacks the cause of the diarrhea. Mix 1 teaspoon in 7 ounces of water and 1 ounce of milk. Take throughout the day as needed. You can also mix 1-2 teaspoon of carob with a creamy rice cereal, a little honey or 1 cup of warm milk. Great for infants in a bottle.

WARNING: Do not give children under one year honey or cow's milk.

Activated Charcoal–Detoxifies the stomach and intestines and absorbs the toxins or bacteria in the stomach that causes diarrhea. Burn toast, then scrape burnt part off and mix in a little milk several times daily. The best form is activated charcoal capsules or tablets (ask your pharmacist or health food store for these). A little of the powder form is best for babies in a small amount of food or fluid.

Bananas–Neutralizes and absorbs the toxins that are causing the diarrhea. Use fresh bananas and either chew them well or mash them up.

Barley Water–Absorbs the toxins. Soak or steep 1-2 teaspoons of barley grain. Strain off water and give 1-2 ounces as needed to small babies. Adults take 1 cup as needed.

Cinnamon, Garlic, or Peppermint Oil–These are particularly good for dysentery, colitis, cholera, and diverticulosis. Make a tea by putting 10-20 drops of the oil in a cup of hot water or juice, drinking 2-3 times a day. Garlic oil is great for Montezuma's Revenge.

SINGLE HERBAL REMEDIES

Catnip or Comfrey Root–Works well for colitis or dysentery and diarrhea in general. Catnip is especially effective for children. Make a tea with either herb.

Myrrh–For chronic diarrhea take 1/2 teaspoon as needed. You may also make a tea.

Bayberry–This is great for colitis, and dysentery or general diarrhea. Make a tea.

COMMERCIALLY PREPARED REMEDIES

Herbs: Kalmin (antispasmodic extract); Ex-Stress Formula capsules or extract (Calms the nervous system.); Cal-Silica Formula (Natural calcium that supports the nervous system.); IF Formula (for inflammation) (Nature's Way); Rescue Remedy (for shock, fright, or trauma) (Bach); or, liquid trace mineral (Take 1/2 ounce in 4-6 ounces of juice 2-4 times daily. Great for dysentery, irritated colon and keeps electrolytes from dropping too low during diarrhea and fever.).

Homeopathic: Nausea; Teething; Flu; or, Emotional (Natra-Bio); Diarrhea; Colic; or, Teething (Hylands); or, Colic; Cold & Flu; or, Teething (Medicine from Nature).

DIZZINESS

Like diarrhea, dizziness is a symptom and not a condition per se. It can be due to many different causes such as something that doesn't agree with an individual, high or low blood pressure, overstressed adrenals, low blood sugar, anemia, B-12 deficiency, colds, flu, reactions to medication, fear, shock from an accident or emotional stress. If dizziness is accompanied by nausea see "Nausea" as well.

> **WARNING:** If symptoms persist after trying one of the simple remedies for a few days, please refer to your doctor for a complete physical.

ACTION

Try to determine the basic cause and then use one of the following remedies. If dizziness is from a medication reaction see your doctor. If you have a history of blood pressure or blood sugar problems use one of the remedies listed below until you can check with your doctor.

KITCHEN REMEDIES

Apple Cider Vinegar, Apple, or Grape Juice–Drink 4 ounces of any of these diluted with warm water. They assist in balancing electrolytes, blood sugar, and settling the stomach. If you use apple cider vinegar, add some honey.

Sage–Settles and balances system and is good for nausea. Make a tea.

Honey or Hard Candy–Hold a small amount of honey in the mouth and let it dissolve slowly. Helps to increase blood sugar. Try to use the natural candy found in health food stores and suck on them if you begin to fell light headed. Keep candy at your desk, in your glove compartment, purse or pocket.

Cloves–Cloves offset nausea. Steep 1 tablespoon of regular, whole cloves, or, 1 teaspoon of powder or crushed cloves about 3 minutes in pint of water. Strain, may add honey and drink as needed.

Garlic–Helps regulate the blood pressure and circulation. Use freshly chopped or squeezed garlic. Mix 1/2-1 tablespoon of garlic in juice or tea.

Raisins–Keep a small box in the car, purse, briefcase, or in desk. This is a natural sweetener that helps if your blood sugar drops.

SINGLE HERBAL REMEDIES

Chamomile–Soothes and calms the body's systems. Make a tea.

Peppermint or Spearmint–Calms and balances the nervous system. Make a tea.

Rose Hips–The high vitamin C content of this herb allows it to help in cases of general debility and exhaustion, and thus dizziness caused by this. Make a tea.

Valerian or Skullcap–Either one of these remedies calms and feeds the nerves. Make a tea

Catnip or Lemon Grass–These herbs soothes and balances the nervous system. Make a tea. Natural sweetener is optional.

COMMERCIALLY PREPARED HERBAL REMEDIES

Herbs: Kalmin (anti-spasmodic extract); PC Formula (Balances the blood sugar.); Fem-Mend Formula or Change-O-Life (Balances female hormones.); Adren-Aid (Balances adrenals, immune system and blood pressure, if too low.); Cal-Silica Formula (natural calcium for nerves); Motion Mate Formula (for motion sickness); Rescue Remedy (for shock and trauma) (Bach); or, Liquid Trace Mineral (Take about 1/2 ounce in 4-6 ounces of juice 2-3 times daily as electrolytes may have dropped out of the system especially if working in extreme heat or emotions are extreme.). You may also try various natural vegetable herbal iron tonics and B-12 sublingual.

Homeopathic: Nausea; Emotional; PMS; or, Menopause (Natra-Bio); Cold & Flu; Earache; Menopause; Tension; or, Migraine Headache (Medicine from Nature).

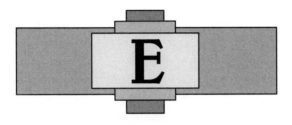

EAR PROBLEMS

Ear problems include pain (throbbing, aching, or sharp) in or around the ear, drainage, ringing, or loss of hearing. Each of these symptoms can be due to many different causes. Pain or hearing loss that is accompanied by fever, fatigue, and malaise is probably an infection. Otitis media or middle ear infection is a common cause of earache among young children. This viral condition may accompany or follow a head cold or flu (see "Colds and Flu"). The risk in not properly treating an ear infection is the development of a secondary bacterial infection. This is the reason why many physicians will prescribe antibiotics for an ear infection. Because antibiotics kill bacteria (not viruses), they do not treat the ear infection itself. If there is discharge from the ear, it may indicate a ruptured ear drum. In most cases, the ear drum will heal on its own with no permanent hearing loss.

Tinnitus, a buzzing, ringing, hissing, roaring, or whistling sound in the ear—in the absence of any outside cause—can be continuous or on again, off again. Because this symptom can occur from almost any ear disorder including infection, ear wax build-up, Meniere's disease, medications, heart disease, anemia, head trauma, or hypertension, it's vital to search for the underlying cause.

Hearing loss and pain also be caused by head injuries, excess ear wax, a tumor, or a foreign object such as a bug stuck in the ear. If hearing loss is chronic, especially in babies or young children, have a physician conduct an auditory test on them.

WARNING: If the ear problems become worse, especially if the person becomes feverish or pain is severe enough to cause crying, call a doctor right away. A discharge from the ear and sudden hearing loss may indicate a punctured ear drum. Call your physician.

ACTION

If ear pain or discomfort appears to be due to an infection, refer to the remedy listed and apply accordingly. If you suspect ear wax is the culprit, use a natural disinfectant and ear bulb from the drugstore to gently clean the ears. Keep on a few minutes before applying remedy or mix suggested remedy with it. Apply the chosen remedy and repeat as needed.

As a general rule, you should not use Q-tips® to clean your ears. This merely clogs your ears up more. The old saying is, "Don't put anything smaller than your elbow in your ear."

KITCHEN REMEDIES

Apple Cider Vinegar Rinse–To remove the toxins, rinse ears with 10 parts of water to 1 part warm apple cider vinegar using an ear bulb. Afterwards place a few diluted drops into ear, plug with cotton, and leave in. Repeat throughout the day or overnight.

Sage–Make a tea adding a 1/4 teaspoon of ginger. For *babies* and *children* steep 1/4-1/2 teaspoon in 1-2 ounces of warm water or juice in a baby bottle or child's cup. *Adults* mix 1/2-1 teaspoon along with the ginger in a cup of warm water or juice. Take this to clean the toxins out of the blood 2-3 times a day as needed.

Garlic–Use fresh garlic that is chopped or squeezed as an antibiotic. Place a drop of olive oil in the ear first, then 1-2 drops of garlic and plug the ear with a little cotton. Apply a garlic poultice around ear after rubbing with a little olive oil. Also use garlic in a tea and add liberally to your diet.

Olive Oil–Place a few drops of warm oil in each ear and plug to soothe the pain and get the toxins out. You can soak some garlic in olive oil for 1-2 hours or overnight and then apply. You can, also, mix an antibiotic oil (a little garlic and good bit of olive oil - 1 to 5 ratio), then drop a few drops of the mixture in each ear. Plug the ear with a little cotton overnight or throughout the day. Repeat as needed.

A neighbor shared with us that while on vacation her ear became infected from swimming. She applied the remedy in this manner and received relief in two hours. She repeated it once and had no more pain.

Cabbage–Place a poultice of warmed finely grated or pulped cabbage around and over ear. Cover with warm cloth and wrap with a towel or scarf. Leave on at least 1-2 hours or overnight. Repeat as needed. Cabbage is a natural antibiotic.

SINGLE HERBAL REMEDIES

Mullein–This is the best of any of the listed remedies for ear infections. It's anti-inflammatory action heals a red, hot ear, especially when used topically. Use 2 warm drops in ears and plug with cotton. In addition, rub some mullein under and around outside of ears. Make a tea.

Clove or Peppermint Oil–Put 2 drops in each ear and plug. Either remedy works as an antiseptic. Make a tea by putting 5-10 drops of the liquid in juice or open 1-2 capsules in a cup of hot water, drinking 2-3 times a day.

Echinacea–This remedy is known as the king of the infection fighters. Make a tea.

Chickweed–Great for cleansing out infections and ulcerations. Make a tea.

Pau d'Arco–You can gently warm the tincture bottle like a baby bottle and place 2 drops in the ear and plug with cotton. Use pau d'arco to fight infections and clean out the toxins in the ear and body. You may also make a tea by putting 10-20 drops of the liquid in juice or open 1-2 capsules in a cup of hot or room temperature water, or in juice. Drink 2-3 times a day.

Sassafras Oil–A good blood purifier and disinfectant. Valuable if ear infection is accompanied by a fever. Mix 5 drops in 1/2 ounce of olive oil and mix well. You may warm it up and place a few drops in each ear and plug, 1-2 times daily.

Thyme Oil–A great infection fighter, especially for an ear infection where there is discharge. Take 5-10 drops of oil in juice or water 2-4 times daily as needed. You may also use 2 drops of warm thyme oil with warm olive oil directly in the ear. Be sure to put olive oil in the ear first, then plug overnight as needed.

OTHER NATURAL TREATMENTS

Ear Bath–Give an ear bulb bath using 1 part warm distilled water to 1 part of apple cider vinegar every seventh day after using drops such as ear garlic oil. If you do not have an ear bulb you can get one from a drug store. Chamomile or goldenseal can be used if ear is inflamed as a rinse. Gently squeeze the warm solution into the ear and let it drain out in the sink or tub. You can leave the herbal residue in, even overnight. Repeat 2-4 hours later, depending on the severity. The next day, rinse ear with 10 parts of distilled or mineral water to 1 part of apple cider vinegar. You can also take other suggested herbs internally to fight infection.

Glycerine–A great solvent that works well with other herbs. This is especially good for an inflamed ear that's red, hot, and aching. Put 2 drops in each ear and plug overnight.

Water Therapy–Place a cool, wet towel around neck while soaking feet in 1 tablespoon of mustard or cayenne pepper dissolved in hot water. This draws the blood away from the head area, reducing the pressure and infection. Herbal drops can be placed in the ears and plugged, if you have any on hand or use any of the suggestions.

Hair Dryer–If your ear problems are caused by swimming, wet weather, a damp basement, a cold, or even sleeping on damp ground when camping, use a dryer on a low setting and blow it in the ear to dry it out.

COMMERCIALLY PREPARED HERBAL REMEDIES

Note: Always wash ears out first. See the Kitchen Remedies section.

Herbs: Kalmin (antispasmodic extract); B&B Formula Extract (Helps clear the ears.); Cayenne-Garlic Formula capsules or drops (Clears general infections.); Fenu-Thyme Formula (for colds and congestion); GL Formula (Cleans glands.); HAS Fast-Acting Formula or HAS Original Formula (free of Pseudoephedrine) (Both cleans the lungs and mucus.); Herbal Influence Formula or Winter Care Formula; or, liquid trace mineral (Take about 1/2 ounces in juice several times daily. Also place 1-2 drops in both ears and plug both ears overnight. Repeat as needed.).

Homeopathic: Earache; Injuries; Cold; Sinus; Flu; Sore Throat; Teething; Teeth & Gums; Candida Yeast; or, Fever (Natra-Bio); Cold & Flu; Earache; Sinusitis or, Teething (Medicine from Nature); Earache; Colic; or, Calms (Hyland). See a homeopath for additional help.

EXHAUSTION

Fatigue or exhaustion can be caused by numerous conditions or situations. We usually associate tiredness with overexertion, insufficient rest or sleep, poor nutrition, obesity, and emotional stress (See "Depression"). Exhaustion can also result from a physical ailment. In this section, I am going to discuss remedies for mental and physical fatigue not due to any discernible disease; exhaustion so great that you cannot push yourself to do or even think about doing anything.

> **WARNING:** If your fatigue doesn't improve after using the following suggestions for one month, see your doctor or a naturopathic physician.

ACTION

To begin with, get plenty of sleep and rest. Rearrange your priorities by cutting down or back on nonessential projects. Do not take on any new activities. Do not feel guilty saying "No" when asked to do something. Improve your diet by eating more grains, vegetables, fruits and drinking more water. Make sure you are getting adequate protein.

Use enemas and soak in a hot herbal bath. Use deep breathing and mild exercise like walking to feed your body more oxygen.

KITCHEN REMEDIES

Juices–Drink fresh juices, hot or cold, made from carrots or grapes with a little apple cider vinegar added. Juices will clean the body of toxins. Selection of fruit is dependent on your own mood and the season of the year.

> **WARNING:** If you're diabetic limit apple and grape juice, as these drinks are high in fruit sugars. Dilute your fruit juices half and half with water.

Sage Tea–This is a very soothing and refreshing drink that can be taken either hot or cold. You may add a single pinch of cayenne, cinnamon, or ginger, or, in combination. Suggest 1-2 cups daily as needed.

Almond Nut Milk–Fill a blender with hot or cold spring water to cover the blades and turn on to high speed. Gradually drop in small amounts of almond nuts, adding more spring water until you have added 2 cups. If you prefer a denser consistency, you may add more nuts. This is a quick and easy way to make a delicious tasting energy drink that is high in vitamins and minerals. For a spicy taste and further help, you can put a pinch of nutmeg, cinnamon, or cayenne into the almond nut milk.

Powerhouse Drink–A great tonic that improves the body's energy and helps clear the mind. Add low-fat goat milk, nut milk, whey milk, buttermilk, yogurt, or coconut milk to cover the blades of a blender and turn on to the high speed setting. Slowly add 1/2-1 cup of almonds; 1 egg and the shell (for calcium); some bananas, apples, or other fruit; 1 tablespoon of wheat germ; 1-3 tablespoons of black strap molasses; and, 1 teaspoon of bran. This will make about 1 quart. Drink 4 ounces three times daily, storing the rest in the refrigerator.

SINGLE HERBAL REMEDIES

Sarsaparilla–Drink 2-3 times daily as a rebuilding tonic. You can mix the sarsaparilla with sage tea using a 50/50 mixture.

Echinacea–Improves the immune system, thus building your body's resistance to infections. Make a tea.

Siberian Ginseng–Known as an energy booster and helps endurance. Make a tea.

OTHER NATURAL TREATMENTS

Enema–To release toxic colon poisons and pressure so you can feel better, mix 1 teaspoon of baking soda or the juice of 1/2 of a **fresh** lemon with seeds strained, into a bag of warm distilled or spring water.

Soak Bath–A great relaxing tonic for the whole body. The heat expands the skin and inner body tissue drawing the toxins to the skins surface and into the water. While filling the tub with hot water add single or combination of herbs desired. Also can use 1-2 cups of epsom salts or 1 cup of aloe vera, apple cider vinegar, cinnamon, or baking soda.

COMMERCIALLY PREPARED HERBAL REMEDIES

Herbs: Adren-Aid (Adrenal support for more energy.); PC Formula (Pancreas support.); Cal-Silica Formula (Natural calcium to enhance nerves and bones.); Change-O-Life or Fem-Mend (Improves energy for the female menstrual system.); H Formula (Strengthens the heart and circulation system.); IF Formula (Supports the immune system.); Liveron (Cleanses the liver.); Red Clover Combination (Cleanses the blood stream.); Ex-Stress (Supports the nervous system.); Naturalax 2, Senna Leaves (Use if bowels feel bloated and sluggish.) (Nature's Way); or, liquid trace minerals (Boosts the body's electrolytes that have dropped from exhaustion.)

Homeopathic: Insomnia; Exhaustion; Emotional (Natra-Bio); Fatigue; PMS; or, Menopause (Medicine from Nature).

EYE PROBLEMS

Complaints about the eyes are varied. They can be vague such as headaches or eye strain or more localized. Pain, redness, swelling, discharge, itching, burning, and irritation all characterize problems of the eyes and eyelids (See "Sty"). These ailments range from structural damage (e.g. retinal detachment) to visual problems, glaucoma and cataracts. Even some systemic diseases may cause eye symptoms.

Because of the complexity of eye problems, I will focus on simple infections of the eye, tear ducts, and eyelids. I will briefly discuss solutions to eye irritation due to environmental exposure.

> **WARNING:** If your eye problem gets worse or does not clear up, see a medical doctor as soon as possible. For severe eye injuries, call 911.

ACTION

Because germs are often introduced by rubbing your eyes, especially if you already have a cold or other infection, **always wash your hands with hot water and a natural soap before you touch the eye area.** You can spread existing eye infections like a sty through hand contact as well.

To prevent this from happening, rinse the eye with a diluted solution of one of the suggested herbal remedies or use a few drops of diluted (50%) of liquid trace mineral or diluted apple cider vinegar (50%) with an eye dropper or eye cup. Liquid trace mineral may give a burning sensation because it is drawing the toxins so fast. This sensation lasts only thirty to sixty seconds. While mowing the lawn a man got a lot of dust and dirt in his eye, he put the liquid mineral in his eye diluted with half water. About five minutes later he washed his eye out with plain water and reapplied the mineral and had no problems with his eye. If the eye burns you may need to dilute the solution even more until it feels a little warm.

If your eyes are chronically itchy, red, and swollen, consider allergies as the source. This could be simply a reaction to cosmetics, lotions, or soap. Or it may be due to hayfever or food allergies. (See "Allergies.")

KITCHEN REMEDIES

Aloe Vera Plant–Cut a small section of leaves, peel to get the gel out, and blend in a little water in a blender. Then spread on a cotton cloth and lay over the eyes for one hour. Aloe vera soothes the eyes and fights infection. Place a few warm drops of aloe juice in each eye 3-4 times daily as needed. This is great for eye redness and irritation from chemicals, fumes, and infection. Use an eye dropper or straw to place a few drops in the eyes or soak with eye cup (see eye bath below).

Castor Oil–Great for reducing swelling. Gently rub some on the eye lids and keeping them closed for 1 hour. Do this several times daily as needed or overnight.

Cod Liver Oil–This may be used for many eye problems for its antiseptic qualities, and high vitamin A and D content. Take 1 teaspoon by itself or in juice 3 times daily. Use especially during the winter months when the air is dried out from heating systems, and if living in a dark, cold winter climate. Also apply some lightly to lids.

Witch Hazel–Take 1/2 teaspoon of this toxin fighter in warm water or juice several times daily as needed. Use 1-2 drops in an eye cup for soaking (see eye bath). You may pour some witch hazel directly onto a cotton ball or cloth, then lay the cloth across closed eyes. This is especially good for bags under the eyes.

Onions–For congested or dry eyes, peel and chop onions, so that tear ducts open. Can keep chopped onions refrigerated in zip bag and re-chop a few times a week, or use in food. You may put an onion by the bed.

Eggs–Beat several fresh egg whites into a foam. Then spread on a linen or cotton cloth and lay over closed eyes for 1 hour (to draw out the infection from the eyes and help the body to heal). Repeat as needed.

SINGLE HERBAL REMEDIES

Echinacea–This remedy works as an antiseptic. Make a tea. May use as an eye soak if needed. Great for conjunctivitis.

Sassafras–The pith from the stem of this plant forms a soothing mucilage in water. It can be used as an eye ointment in cases or irritation and redness.

Goldenseal–Goldenseal is also known as eye root, a fitting description as this herb has been used by third world countries in the treatment of chlamydial trachoma. Soak eyes with the tea to fight infection as described in eye bath below. Make a tea to help boost your immunity.

Burdock–Great for an eye wash and soak to draw out the infection and helps the body to fight the toxins (see eye bath below) that works well for sties. Make a tea.

Mullein–Cleanses the eyes of pus and soothes inflammation. Make a tea. Soak eyes with tea solution in an eye cup.

COMMERCIALLY PREPARED HERBAL REMEDIES

Herbs: Eyebright Combination; Ex-Stress (Supports the nervous system.) (Nature's Way); or liquid trace minerals (Diluted 1/2 and 1/2 to 1 part mineral and 5 parts water. Place 3 to 10 drops in each eye or wet cotton balls and place on eyelids for 45 minutes.)

Homeopathic: Eye Irritation; Exhaustion; Inuries; Pain; Insomnia (Natra-Bio); or Headache (Medicne from Nature).

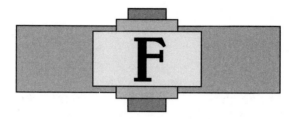

FAINTING

Sudden loss of consciousness or fainting begins when an individual feels weak, nauseated, experiences blurred vision, and starts to sweat and possibly vomit. To the passerby, the person appears pale and perspiring. A diminished flow of blood, and thus oxygen, to the brain, causes a fainting spell. If the person quickly crouches, sits, or lies down, he can often avoid fainting. In either case, fainting or assuming a horizontal position, is the body's corrective measure that sends oxygen rich blood to the head.

Some causes of fainting are sudden shock, bad news, pain, an accident, a blow or fall, high blood pressure, anemia, overtaxed adrenals, or a poor diet. If someone hyperventilates due to excessive worry, this can also cause fainting. Low blood sugar or drugs can sometimes cause loss of consciousness, though unlike true fainting, this occurs over a span of minutes and not immediately.

WARNING: If fainting is from a bad accident, fall, or blow make the injured person comfortable and call for medical help. Check the suggestions below for First Aid help and apply until medics arrive.

ACTION

If you suspect someone is going to faint, having them quickly sit with their head between their legs (see Figure 34), crouch, or lie down may prevent this from happening. If they do faint, make them as comfortable as possible, loosening tight clothing, fanning them, opening windows, elevating their feet and keeping them warm with some kind of covering. If the person remains unconscious you can rub a little of Kalmin (antispasmodic tincture), Rescue Remedy or other aids just inside the mouth, in the navel, or on their hands which will help to bring them around. Also, you may wave ammonia (smelling salts) or a pungent odor like garlic or onion under the nose. Try to determine the cause of fainting, then give herbs from that section, and note any history of fainting.

If fainting is due to a drop in blood sugar, have the person eat something such as raisins, honey, or even some candy. Excessive loss of body fluids and electrolytes can cause fainting spells. This is particularly true on hot summer days for people who work out of doors like crossing guards, policeman, road workers, and door-to-door sales people. Drink more water and use the Liquid Trace Mineral to build up the fluids.

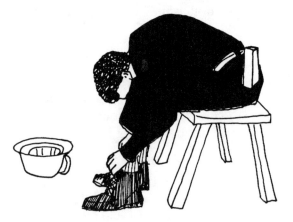

Figure 34 First Aid for Fainting

- If the person feels faint, the initial response might be sitting with the head between the knees.

- Have the victim lie down with the head lower than the feet.

KITCHEN REMEDIES

Cayenne–Cayenne is great in equalizing blood pressure whether from a fall, injury, or emotional shock. If the person is unconscious, apply the mixture on the feet, hands, or chest, however it is best to apply it in the navel. Take 1/4 teaspoon of tincture, powder or 1-2 capsules and work up to 1-2 teaspoons throughout the day. Then 1-2 times daily for maintenance.

Honey–Place a little in the mouth if exhausted or if blood sugar drops.

Grapes or Apples–Drink a little juice or eat the fresh fruit to raise blood sugar.

Herbal Teas–Various teas, such as peppermint and spearmint, are very good in relaxing and supporting the nerves. You can use them either as a single herb tea or in combination. If you have any of these herbs as loose leaves in your kitchen, then brew your own teas.

Apple Cider Vinegar–Take 1/2-1 teaspoon in 6 ounces of cool or hot water or juice adding a little honey. It strengthens the system.

Raisins–Carry a small box in your purse, pocket, or briefcase for emergencies. For a small blood sugar increase, chew a few raisins or a handful until you can eat or feel better.

SINGLE HERBAL REMEDIES

Chamomile–This works as a mild sedative and is helpful when you are experiencing dizziness or nervousness. Make a tea.

Catnip–This is great for dizziness, spasms, nervousness, fevers, or headaches. You can combine with chamomile. Make a tea.

Valerian–This is great for nerves, and particularly for dizziness. Make a tea.

Lemon Grass–A great aid for stress, headaches, and dizziness. Make a tea.

Peppermint Oil–This carminative herb is good for the nausea, and vomiting that may accompany fainting. Take 5-10 drops in a tea form or in a little warm apple juice, sipping slowly until finished. Works best when warm and great when combined with a few drops of elder flower.

COMMERCIALLY PREPARED HERBAL REMEDIES

Herbs: Kalmin (antispasmodic extract); Adren-Aid (Supports adrenal glands and low blood pressure.); PC Formula (Balances pancreas and blood sugar.); Ex-Stress (Supports the nervous system); Fem-Mend or Change-O-Life (menopause); B/P Formula or CapsiCool (Helps blood pressure.) (Nature's Way); Liquid Trace Minerals (Provides electrolytes and helps keep the body in balance from fainting.); or, Rescue Remedy (for shock and trauma) (Bach).

Homeopathic: Raw Adrenal; Raw Pancreas; Emotional; Injuries; or, Menopause (Natra-Bio.); Fatigue; or, Menopause (Medicine from Nature).

FEVER

We have been taught that normal body temperature is 98.6° F. However, the truth is that body temperature can vary widely among individuals (between 96.6 and 99.4). There are also normal variations in body temperature throughout the day. The way you take your temperature can influence a reading. Most information on fevers is based on oral readings. If you take a temperature under the arm (call axillary temperature), it is about one degree lower than an oral reading. A rectal temperature is approximately one degree higher. Don't assume you can judge a fever by laying your hand on someone's forehead or face. Research shows that even trained professionals are unable to do this.

However, when this temperature exceeds 100° F and is accompanied by other symptoms, you will want to treat the person. Chills and night sweats may accompany a fever and help doctors identify the reason for the fever. In children, fevers tend to be higher. As people age, this fever response diminishes.

Fevers occur in both infectious and noninfectious conditions. A fever may be due to drugs, trauma, a heart attack, rheumatoid arthritis, or dehydration especially among infants and the elderly. However, this section will focus on fevers due to infections or food poisoning.

Most of us are conditioned to treat fevers with aspirin or other medicines. However, an elevated body temperature is the body's way of fighting an infection. Take this into consideration before administering a fever reducing remedy. It is more prudent to treat the underlying infection. You should also ensure that the patient's fluid intake is adequate. Dehydration can be a serious problem. If the fever causes discomfort such as aching joints, use one of the following fever-reducing remedies.

If the fever continues for more than three days and is accompanied by other symptoms, see your doctor. Tell him the nature of the fever (if its continuous or accompanied by chills and night sweats) and other symptoms. If you suspect food poisoning, see the section on "Food Poisoning."

> **WARNING:** If your newborn develops a fever during his first few months of life, see your doctor immediately. If the patient's body temperature climbs due to heat exhaustion, overexertion in hot weather or prolonged exposure to a Jacuzzi or sauna, rush him to the hospital immediately.

ACTION

An enema is the quickest way to reduce a high fever. Be sure to take in plenty of water, soups, herbal teas, and juices to prevent dehydration. For adults, put 1/2 tablespoon of Liquid Trace Minerals in their drinks several times daily to help keep electrolytes balanced during the fever and to offset dehydration.

KITCHEN REMEDIES

Apple Cider Vinegar–This clears toxins out of the system and opens pores. Drink 1/2-1 teaspoon in a cup of hot water. After drinking it down, cover up for warmth and sweat out the toxins.

Lemon Juice–Squeeze 1/2 of a lemon in a cup of hot water. Drink and cover up. This aids sweating to break fever.

Ginger–Brew and drink this tea for fevers from colds and flu. Ginger is a diaphoretic meaning it causes you to sweat.

Peppermint/Spearmint–This tea works for chills and fevers as well as colds and the flu. If you have any elder flower add a few drops to the tea, especially if you need to break a high fever. Either one of these teas are great in enemas.

Garlic or Onion–These vegetables fight the infection and increase perspiration to get rid of the toxins. Chop or juice about 1/2 teaspoon of each, then soak in 2 ounces of apple cider vinegar for a few minutes. Next, add 1/2 teaspoon of the mixture to hot water, tea, or juice. Drink as needed. You can also use garlic oil.

Cloves–Best to use fresh cloves to fight the toxins, if you have some, and steep 1 teaspoon for a few minutes, strain, add honey to sweeten, if necessary, and drink as needed. You can also use 10-20 drops of clove oil.

Barley–Good for high fevers and may be used in a fever reducing enema. Boil about 1 cup's worth in linen, or cotton cloth for about 30 minutes in 1-1 1/2 quarts of water or strain the barley out after it cooks. Drink 1/2-1 cup every 1-2 hours as needed.

SINGLE HERBAL REMEDIES

Echinacea–A great all around antibiotic that is safe to use for babies. Make a tea by putting 10-20 drops of the liquid in juice (2 to 5 for *babies* in a bottle) or open 1-2 capsules in a cup of hot or room temperature water, or in juice. Drink 2-3 times a day.

Lemon Grass–Great anti-fever remedy that works well for stress and colds. Make a tea.

Red Raspberry–Good for fevers from various viruses or food poisoning. You may add red raspberry drops to spearmint, peppermint, or catnip tea as an antispasmodic to relax the body. Make a tea.

Boneset–To break high fevers take 1-2 teaspoons of the tincture in a cup of hot water and take every 1-2 hours as needed. To regulate the fever take 20-30 drops. Great for severe fevers, chills and deep bone ache. Best as warm tea which you can add drops to warm water or warm apple juice. Like the red raspberry herb, you can add boneset knit to catnip, peppermint, or spearmint tea as an antispasmodic.

Elder Flowers–Use as a hot tea (diaphoretic) to break fevers. Make a tea. You can also add this herb to peppermint tea or use in a hot soak bath (see below).

Feverfew–As its name suggests, this herb is good for all different types of fevers. Make a tea.

Yarrow–Terrific for fevers from measles, colds, or flu. Make a tea. This herb combines well with elder flower or boneset.

OTHER NATURAL TREATMENTS

Soak Bath–The heat from a hot bath opens the skin's pores thus allowing elimination of toxins. While filling the tub with hot water add single or combination of herbs desired. Tinctured or liquid teas are very good here. Also, use 1-2 cups of epsom salts or 1 cup of: aloe vera, apple cider vinegar, or baking soda for a soak bath.

If the person is too hot due to fever they may need a cold water or an ice bath or an alcohol sponge bath. This helps to keep temperature down until you can get professional assistance.

Enema–Mix 1 teaspoon of baking soda or the juice of 1/2 of a **fresh** lemon with seeds strained, into a bag of warm distilled or spring water. Use in an enema.

COMMERCIALLY PREPARED HERBAL REMEDIES

Herbs: GL Formula (for gland swelling); Breath-Aid Formula (for respiratory infections); Fenu-Thyme Formula (Cleanses lung congestion.); Winter Care Formula or Herbal Influence; or, Kalmin (An antispasmodic that is good for Scarlet or Spotted fever. Take 5-8 drops in juice as needed.) (Nature's Way).

Homeopathic: Fever; Flu; Teething; Cold; Sore Throat; or, Earache (Natra-Bio); or, Earache; Cold & Flu; Teething; or, Sinusitis (Medicine from Nature).

FOOD POISONING

There are times when we are sent to bed for a day with an upset stomach. Most people call this the 24-hour flu. In fact, it's more likely food poisoning.

Typically, symptoms appear suddenly as nausea, vomiting, diarrhea, stomach cramps, and loss of appetite. Exhaustion, muscle aches, fever, and a general ill feeling may also be present. Excessive vomiting and diarrhea can lead to dehydration and shock. Symptoms usually last for a few hours in mild cases, a couple of days in more severe instances.

Traveler's diarrhea or Montezuma's revenge is usually due to E. coli, bacterial toxins, and some viruses. Salmonella, a common contaminant of poultry and eggs, can also cause illness. Botulism, from the toxin of Clostridium botulinum, can develop from poisoned food or infected wounds. Home canned foods are often the culprit behind botulism.

Other causes of food poisoning include poisonous mushrooms and other plants, poisonous fish or shellfish and chemically contaminated foods. (See "Poisons.")

WARNING: Symptoms of botulism include the usual food poisoning signs followed by dry mouth, double vision, weakness, and sometimes paralysis. If you suspect someone has botulism, transport him to the hospital immediately. If someone has ingested a poisonous plant or mushroom, call your local Poison Control Center or hospital.

If someone has food poisoning symptoms that are severe or last for more than a day, call your doctor.

ACTION

PREVENTION Unfortunately, spoiled food can't always be detected by taste, appearance, or smell. So when in doubt, throw it out. Unsanitary handling of food, such as using a cutting board or knife contaminated with raw poultry to chop vegetables, can cause Salmonella poisoning. Leaving perishable food unrefrigerated for several hours, can also cause spoiling. Protein foods such as meat, and milk and eggs are especially prone to contamination. Be sure to adequately cook or heat food to prevent botulism and other forms of food poisoning. If you plan to can foods, make sure you follow directions carefully. If you have an open sore on your hand, cover it with a bandaid or have someone else cook.

TREATMENT If someone has already been poisoned by food, try to determine the source and throw any leftovers out. Keep the person warm and comfortable while having them take the suggested remedies. If the food poisoning is from a restaurant or a friend's house, contact them immediately to tell them what has happened.

KITCHEN REMEDIES

Sage–Make a tea to clean the body of toxins.

Spearmint or Peppermint Teas–Either of these teas will settle the bowels and the stomach from nausea. If you think that botulism is the cause, this remedy is very good. (Do this while awaiting medical help. Always transport cases of botulism to the hospital immediately.) In addition, either is good to drink before or after throwing up.

Ginger–Fresh ginger root or powder works well for food poisoning and dysentery. Make a tea.

Baking Soda–In 4 ounces of warm water mix 1/4 teaspoon of baking soda and sip over 30 minutes while sitting up. Repeat the use of this antacid as needed.

WARNING: Unless your doctor supervises you, do not administer to children under 5 years old. Don't take more than 1/2 tsp. 8 times a day if you're under 60 years old or 1/2 tsp. 4 times a day if you're over 60 in a 24-hour period. Don't take this maximum dose for more than 2 weeks. Don't use baking soda if you're on a sodium restricted diet.

Activated Charcoal–Stir in 1/2 teaspoon of powdered charcoal in a cup of hot water, then drink to neutralize the stomach acids. Honey may be added to sweeten if desired. You may follow this drink with a little juice or an herb tea. Repeat as needed. You can purchase this from a drugstore or health food store.

Garlic–Use fresh garlic that has been squeezed, grated, or chopped to clean the body of toxins. Then mix in a cup of hot tea, herbal teas, or room temperature juice. You can also use garlic oil.

Apple Cider Vinegar–Mix 1 teaspoon of the antiseptic apple cider vinegar in 8 ounces of warm water and sip 4 ounces every 1-2 hours as needed.

Carbonated water or soda–When you have no other remedies, sip slowly, 4 ounces of any of these sodas every 1-2 hours as needed. The carbonation helps to relieve gases. So, burp freely.

Coffee–This is an old Italian trick to settle the stomach after eating heavy meals. It works as an antacid. Drink a strong cup of coffee without any sugar or cream. Repeat as needed.

Blessed Thistle or Cornflower–Another ancient remedy used by the Native Americans of the plains to counteract various toxins; mix 1/2-1 teaspoon in a cup of hot water, adding honey to sweeten is optional.

Salt–Occasionally, one may need to rid the system of the toxins by inducing vomiting. Using salt as an emetic by drinking 1 tablespoon in 6-8 ounces of warm water. Save some salt water to soothe the stomach after throwing up.

SINGLE HERBAL REMEDIES

Red Raspberry–This remedy eases the diarrhea that is part of food poisoning, Montezuma's revenge, or any other stomach and bowel problem. Take 15-20 drops in a cup of water, or 2 capsules every 1-2 hours.

Sarsaparilla–Great as a poison antidote and works as a tonic to purify the blood. Take 1-2 teaspoons or 2 capsules or make a tea drink every 1-2 hours as needed.

Sassafras–A powerful blood purifier that destroys some microorganisms and takes care of systemic infections. Take 1/2-1 teaspoon of tincture or 2 capsules. You can also make a tea and drink every 1-2 hours as needed. For the best of both, combine sassafras with sarsaparilla in equal parts.

Fennel–This is a good soothing stomach aid which works as an antiseptic. Make a tea. **WARNING:** Large amounts can disturb the nervous system.

Gentian–This is one of the best stomach tonics that is high in iron and aids the weak and convalescing patients. Make a tea.

Plantain or Burdock Root–Both of these are powerful remedies that cleanse the blood. Plantain also treats diarrhea. Put 10-15 drops in hot water or non-citrus juice or take 2 capsules 3-4 times daily, or as needed.

OTHER NATURAL TREATMENTS

Induce Vomiting–To empty your stomach of the poisoned food, stick your finger to the back of your throat to induce the gag reflex and vomiting. Be gentle when you do this so as not to damage your throat.

Ipecac Syrup–Use this to induce vomiting. It is especially good for small children to expel poisons. This may be acquired from a drug store. Follow the directions on the bottle or call your doctor.

Enema–You can use buttermilk or cultured yogurt which help counter the bad bacteria. If you don't have either one of these, mix

1 teaspoon of baking soda or the juice of 1/2 of a **fresh** lemon with seeds strained, into a bag of warm distilled or spring water. Use these in an enema.

COMMERCIALLY PREPARED REMEDIES

Herbs: Kalmin (anti-spasmodic); Naturalax 1, 2, or 3, Aloelax or Senna Leaves; or, Liveron (Cleanses liver and gall bladder.) (Nature's Way).

Homeopathic: Nausea; Headache & Pain; Indigestion; Laxative; or, Flu (Natra-Bio); Indigestion & Gas; Colic; or, Headache (Medicine from Nature); or, Colic; or, Diarrhea (Hylands).

FROSTBITE, AND OTHER COLD INJURIES

Exposure to the cold, whether it's from falling into an icy river, being inadequately dressed in winter weather or getting caught in the rain on a cool day for several hours without a warm refuge, can be dangerous. You can distinguish frostbite from other cold injuries by the cold, white, hard appearance of the area which turns blotchy red and swollen upon rewarming. The person initially tells you he can't feel anything in the frostbit region, however, once it begins to heat up the area can become very painful.

A more superficial cold injury, called frostnip, occurs when the cold is also damp. Here the face, ears, hands, or feet are usually involved and look like frostbite at first glance. However, a day or two later peeling and even blistering may happen and cause a minor cause of cold sensitivity.

Chilblains is a more severe damp cold condition. Feet, hands and ears swell and turn pale. They feel numb and clammy or will itch and burn. Sores can develop. Long term, the area becomes more susceptible to cold, hypersensitive, swells and sweats easily because of nerve and blood vessel damage.

Finally, there's hypothermia which literally means a lower body temperature. If severe, this condition can be life threatening. You've probably heard stories about people who have gone for hikes and been found wandering aimlessly, unable to find their way home. Left untreated, exposure can result in lethargy, confusion, hallucinations, and unconsciousness. Breathing and heartbeat can slow down and eventually stop.

All of these conditions are more likely if a person is tired hungry, drunk, or wearing wet clothes. Those who have heart disease, or are very young or very old are also more susceptible. Windchill can also exaggerate cold conditions and cold injuries.

WARNING: In severe cases of frostbite or prolonged cold exposure, call for an ambulance immediately. In the meantime carry out the following first aid suggestions.

DO NOT give the patient alcohol.

DO NOT allow the person to walk on frostbitten feet. The exception to this rule, is if the person must walk to help.

DO NOT rewarm the affected area first.

DO NOT let the person sit near a fire or other intense heat.

ACTION

Contrary to popular belief, using ice or snow is not a safe way to treat a cold injury. Do not rub or use direct heat on a person with frostbite, frostnip, or chilblains. Handle the injured area very gently. Instead, cover the frozen body part and person with a dry blanket or clothes. Get him inside as quickly as possible and rapidly warm him up with a lukewarm—**not hot**—bath. Because frostbitten areas are often numb, the patient will not be able to tell if something is too hot. Make sure your bath doesn't exceed 105° F. Stop warming frostbite when the skin becomes flushed.

After the bath, cleanse the affected area with water and natural soap and pat dry with clean towels. If fingers or toes are affected, place dry, sterile gauze between these digits. Elevate frostbitten parts and do not break blisters that may form.

If a bath isn't available, wrap the affected areas in blankets. Do not remove clothing if it is stuck to the skin. Wait until the skin warms up, then the clothes will loosen by themselves. Dress the person warmly. Have him drink some warm soup or tea if he is conscious and not vomiting.

If exposure is the problem, carry out above suggestions. In addition to these, remove all wet clothes and anything else that may constrict circulation. If you are not near proper facilities, frostbitten areas can be warmed on a companion, especially against his stomach or under his arms.

KITCHEN REMEDIES

Aloe Vera Plant–Cut enough leaves to cover the frostbite and put in a blender. Add 1/4 teaspoon of cayenne pepper and enough warm olive oil to cover the blades, then mix on high speed. Warm the mixture up slightly and apply gently over the exposed area about every 1-2 hours until the skin improves or you receive medical assistance. Refrigerate the extra mixture and warm as needed.

Cinnamon, Ginger, and Sage–Put a 1/2 teaspoon of each, especially cinnamon, into a warm cup of tea and drink it all down. This slowly improves the body heat and circulation. In addition, you may rub the tea over the frostbite after some tea or soup has been drunk.

Lemon-Cayenne Rub–First, gently rub warm lemon juice onto the frostbite. Next, combine 1 teaspoon of powdered cayenne pepper with 1 pint of warm olive oil and mix well. Then gently rub the oil over the frostbite and cover it to keep the heat in. This remedy brings gets the blood moving, brings warmth to the frostbite and keeps the skin from further damage. You can also use cayenne oil. Take cayenne oil or powder as tea form as well.

WARNING: Do not apply cayenne to open sores or blisters.

Olive, Vegetable, or Wheat Germ Oil–If you do not have the ingredients for the lemon-cayenne rub, then you can gently rub in the area with any of these warmed oils. Repeat every 1-2 hours, keeping warm until better or get to medical help. Keeps the skin from becoming more damaged.

SINGLE HERBAL REMEDIES

Echinacea–This supports the immune system to fight off cold and chill factors. Make a tea.

Siberian Ginseng–Strengthens immune system and stamina. Make a tea.

OTHER NATURAL TREATMENTS

Vitamin A or E (100-400 IU)–Hold the perle in the hands to warm it up, then puncture it and put a few drops of oil on the worse areas as needed. In addition take 1-2 perles several times daily.

> **WARNING:**   Do not take more than 50,000 IU of vitamin A for extended periods of time unless under supervision of a doctor.

COMMERCIALLY PREPARED HERBAL REMEDIES

Herbs: Cayenne-Garlic Formula is for extreme frostbite or if a person is close to frozen. If the person is unconscious rub a few warm drops in the navel or mix the formula with either warm water or warm vegetable oil, applying to the fingers and toes. When the person can sit up give 1/2 of a capsule mixed in a warm herbal tea or water with a little honey for taste. Sip slowly until the body warms up. When you are warmer and can swallow, you can take the other 1/2 of the capsule by mouth. If you cannot swallow the rest of the capsule, then mix it in another cup of warmer to hotter herbal tea. Do so until you get warmer and stronger with better circulation. Then can take 1 capsule every 2-4 hours to improve circulation and warmth.

Other herbs are: Adren-Aid Formula (Increases and supports adrenal energy to the body, heart, and circulation.); IF Formula (Supports immune system to fight off cold and chill factors.); Winter Care Formula (Strengthens and protects lungs.) or Herbal Influence Formula; Breath-Aid (for respiratory problems and colds); Ex-Stress (Supports the nervous system.); Echinacea Combination (Supports the immune system.); or, Rescue Remedy (for sudden shock and trauma) (Bach).

Homeopathic: Injuries; Cold; Earache; Flu; or, Emotional (Natra-Bio); or, Cold & Flu; or, Earache (Medicine from Nature).

FUNGUS

Fungus is a general term that refers to yeasts and molds. This lower form of plant life plays an important role in our lives. It provides us with food like mushrooms and as baking yeast for bread, its brewers's yeast allows us to make alcohol and we use some types to manufacture medicines such as antibiotics.

However, there are a few forms that are bothersome to humans. (See "Yeast Infections.") One group of fungus, commonly called ringworm, causes superficial infections; it's notorious for invading various body parts. When one of these fungi blacken a toe or fingernail, its called ringworm of the nails or onychomycosis. Nails become thick and dull. This is a long term and usually difficult condition to treat.

If this occurs on the skin in the genital area, we label it jock itch. Itching and scratching causes further skin irritation. Recurrence is common and is frequently worse in the summer. Foot fungus is usually referred to as athlete's foot. It's commonly found between toes and on the sole of the foot.

This fungal villain will also attack the body's skin in general, thus becoming ringworm of the body. You can distinguish this condition by its round, red rings.

ACTION

These fungal infections are difficult to identify without professional help. Your doctor needs to scrape the rash and look at its cells under a microscope or attempt to grow the fungus in the laboratory before a positive diagnosis can be made. The following remedies, while generally safe, may not be effective if you're not sure you have a fungal condition.

Before using a disinfectant and suggested aid, wash the fungus with a natural soap and water, drying well.

For athlete's foot or jock itch, change socks or underwear daily. Since washing doesn't always completely kill the offending fungus, try ironing your socks and underwear between wearings. After applying a selected remedy, you may cover the hands or feet with clean, natural cloth gloves or socks, preferably white.

Since persistent or repeated fungal infections are a sign that your immune system is not functioning at its best, work on improving your overall health by including more fresh fruits and vegetables, whole grains, legumes, dried beans, fish and skinless poultry in your diet. Drink at least six glasses of a day water to flush out the toxins in your body and to keep your bowels open.

KITCHEN REMEDIES

Aloe Vera–Slice a piece of a plant, then tape it to the infected area to fight the toxins and soothe the skin. You can also blend some of the plant into a paste with a little olive oil. Apply paste, then cover it by taping it to a cotton cloth or bandage. You can also cover the feet or hands with clean, white gloves or socks for athlete's feet. Aloe vera is a natural antibiotic and soothes the irritation. Keep the extra mixture refrigerated and apply as needed.

Garlic, Cabbage, Onion, or Potato–Freshly crush or finely mince any of the recommended vegetables to work as infection fighters and aids in healing. To protect the skin, apply a light coating of vegetable, olive, or wheat germ oil first before you place the vegetables. Also, mix a vegetable in water or a little juice to drink, or make a poultice to use overnight. You can also apply garlic oil alone from the health food store, or take in a tea.

Antifungal Paste–Mix a 1/2 tablespoon of sage, 1/4 teaspoon of cinnamon, 1/4 teaspoon of cayenne with enough olive oil to make a paste. Apply to the fungus and cover with a clean cotton cloth, socks or gloves. Reapply as needed after washing and disinfecting area. If this irritates your skin, try the paste without cayenne.

Olive or Wheat Germ Oil–Apply a few drops of either natural antifungal oil to the fungus 1-2 times daily, or rub either oil onto the fungus with a disinfected finger or cotton. You may also add a little vitamin E (100-400 IU) to the oil.

Castor Oil–This suffocates and expels the fungus. Rub over the fungus 1-2 times a day, leaving on overnight. Wash the area once a week unless your are expelling dead skin.

Lemon–This citrus fruit acts as a natural antiseptic. Dilute 1 part lemon to 3 parts water and apply with cotton cloth to infected area. If the solution burns, dilute it with more water.

Figs, Prunes, or Raisins–Mash a combination or singular fruit up and use as a poultice. All of these are antifungal.

Corn Starch, Powder–Make an antiseptic paste by mixing a little water or vegetable oil in with the corn starch and apply to the area with a disinfected finger or cotton. Cover the area with a clean cotton cloth, gloves, or socks.

SINGLE HERBAL REMEDIES

With any of the following herbal remedies you may foment the fungal infection as well as take internally. For fomentation, apply the warm oil or liquid with a cloth or directly onto the affected area.

Keep moist by adding the oil or liquid to the cloth or redampen cloth by immersion and reapply.

Black Walnut–The extract is great as an antifungal for various related conditions. Make a tea

Chickweed–Use either the extract or ointment an antifungal and to fight the toxins for various skin fungus. Apply directly to the fungus. Make a tea.

Pau d'Arco–The extract combats various fungi and parasites. Apply directly to the infected area or take as a tea.

Myrrh–A powerful antiseptic that can be spread, undiluted, over the fungus 3-4 times daily or overnight. Cover the area with a clean cloth, socks, or gloves. Also, take 6 drops in a cup of warm water or juice 3-4 times daily.

Figwort–This is great for various skin diseases that cause itching and irritation. Make a tea.

> **WARNING:** Don't take figwort if you have tachycardia or an unusually rapid heartbeat.

OTHER NATURAL TREATMENTS

Soak Bath–The heat draws toxins to the skin's surface. While filling the tub with hot water suited to your body temperature, add the single or combination of herbs desired. Tinctured or liquid teas are very good here. In addition, you can use 1-2 cups of epsom salts, 1 cup of: aloe vera, apple cider vinegar, or baking soda. Be careful that you thoroughly dry the infected area.

Vitamin E (100-400 IU)–Place a few drops of the liquid vitamin on the affected area a couple times daily to aid healing. Also, you can add a little wheat germ oil or puncture a vitamin A perle and apply either to the fungus along with the vitamin E. Take 1-2 perles of vitamin E 2-3 times daily (no more than 400 IU of vitamin E daily).

COMMERCIALLY PREPARED HERBAL REMEDIES

Herbs: BF&C (Rebuilds bone, flesh and cartilage); Black or, Comfrey ointment (rash and fungus healers); Red Clover Combination (Purifies blood stream.); IF Formula (immune support); PARA-X capsules, or PARA-VF (fungus and parasite cleansers); Naturalax 1, 2, or 3, or Aloelax (Moves toxic bowels) (Nature's Way); or, liquid trace mineral (Great fungus fighter. Take 1/2 ounces in juice 2-3 times daily. Also, soak hands or feet in a pan or use a moistened cloth or cotton to dab the remedy on the fungus several times daily.)

Homeopathic: Mycosode (Works on 28 different fungi.); Mycological Immune Stimulator (Professional Health); or, Candida Yeast; or, Detoxification (Natra-Bio.).

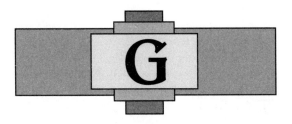

GALLSTONES

Gallstones are a common condition occurring in approximately one-tenth of all Americans. This ailment is an example of a condition caused, or at least provoked, by unhealthy eating. A low fiber, high-fat diet has been proven to promote gallstones. Food allergies may also contribute to this disease.

Most people with gallstones have no or only mild symptoms such as gas, occasional nausea, vomiting, cramps, bloating, an intolerance to some foods and a sour brackish, foul taste in the mouth. However, others may also experience gallbladder attacks, also called biliary colic, that are minor or severe. This gripping pain usually occurs in or under the right front ribs and liver area, sometimes extending to the tip of right shoulder blade. It frequently wakes the person up at night or happens after eating too many greasy fried foods.

Gallstones are composed of either pure cholesterol, all minerals, or pure pigment or calcium bilirubinate. However, the most common stones are mixed types which contain cholesterol, bile pigments, and calcium and bile salts. Sometimes gallstones can pass easily and at other times they are too large to pass on through the gallbladder or bile ducts and become stuck causing severe pain. Standard medical treatment for gallstones is either medication to dissolve the gallstones or removal of the gallbladder.

WARNING: If fever and gallbladder pain as described above persist call the doctor right away.

ACTION

If you have a gallbladder attack, stop eating solid foods, especially fatty ones, to give the gallbladder a rest. Instead drink apple juice to keep the bowels open and apply the following remedies until you can check with a doctor.

KITCHEN REMEDIES

Apple Juice–Drink about 6 ounces of warm apple juice every hour while using other remedies below. It softens the stones while the other aids may give relief.

Gallbladder Prevention–To help prevent a congested gall bladder, drink 1 glass of apple juice or apple cider vinegar about 6 times daily for 3 days. During this time you can water fast or eat soft, light food. On the third night drink the lemon and olive oil mixture (see below) and go to bed. Repeat this about two to three times a year.

Another prevention is that you may add oil to 1/2 teaspoon of sage and 1/4 teaspoon of cinnamon in a cup of hot water and drink 2-3 times a day.

Parsley Leaf–Put a hand full of fresh parsley cut in short pieces in a quart of hot water, simmering 5 minutes. Strain and drink 1 warm cup of this tea 3 times a day.

WARNING: Very large doses of parsley leaf can cause nerve damage, bleeding in the gut, and problems with the liver. Don't use if you're pregnant.

Sage–Make a tea to clean out the toxins adding either singularly or both 1/4 teaspoon of ginger or cinnamon.

SINGLE HERBAL REMEDIES

Barberry–Since this is bitter by itself, use 10-20 drops with other tinctures or teas, like mint. Works on sluggish liver and gallbladder conditions. Especially good for inflamed gallbladders and gallstones.

Dandelion–A great help for gallstones, enlarged liver, hepatitis, jaundice, and cleans the blood. The roasted root makes a good coffee substitute. Make a tea.

Fennel–Use this for jaundice, obstructions of liver, gall bladder, and spleen. Make a tea, drink one or two cups a day.

> **WARNING:** Very large amounts of fennel can disturb the nervous system.

Parsley Root–Helps with problems of jaundice, stones, and liver or spleen obstructions. (See "Parsley leaf."). Make a tea. You can make a great tea combining 5-10 drops of parsley with 5-10 drops of wild yam in a pint of water. Drink 1 cup throughout the day.

Wild Yam Extract–Mix this tea in cool water, not hot. Make a tea by putting 10-20 drops of the liquid in juice or open 1-2 capsules in a cup of hot water, drinking 2-3 times a day. This antispasmodic is great for bilious colic (spasms due to gallbladder problems).

White Oak Bark Extract–If you have gallstones, this is great because of its anti-inflammatory action. Make a tea.

COMMERCIALLY PREPARED HERBAL REMEDIES

Herbs: Liveron (Supports liver and gall bladder.); Kalmin (antispasmodic); Cal-Silica Formula (Calcium balance improves the liver function.); Red Clover Combination (Cleanses bloodstream.); Naturalax 1,2, or 3, or, Aloelax (Either cleanses the toxic bowels.); PARA-X Formula (for parasites) (Nature's Way); Liquid Trace Mineral (A great tonic taken with 1/2 ounce of mineral in about 4-6 ounces of vegetable or fruit juice. Drink several times daily.); or, Rescue Remedy (for shock and trauma) (Bach).

Homeopathic: Nausea; Laxative; Emotional; Candida Yeast; Raw Liver; Detoxification; Indigestion; Headache & Pain; or, Pain (Natra-Bio); Indigestion & Gas; or, Colic (Medicine from Nature); or, Gall Bladder (BHI).

GOUT

Gout is a common disease that has been known since antiquity. Well-fed men with straining waistcoats feasting on spirits and rich foods while nursing a sore, big toe propped up on a stool is the historical picture of gout. To some extent, this portrayal is true.

This ailment is due to excessive uric acid in bodily fluids which settles in the joints, tendons, kidneys, and other tissues. It manifests as unusual soreness or tenderness, swelling, and hot throbbing pain in the joints, most often at night. About half of people with gout have the classically sore big toe.

Attacks of gout typically occur after overindulging in food or alcohol, or wearing ill-fitting shoes. Surgery, trauma, infections, fatigue, stress, and some drugs also provoke an attack. If long enough, some attacks are accompanied by fevers, chills, and an ill feeling. Gout attacks can last from a few days to weeks, although the person is otherwise without symptoms. Men are predominantly afflicted by gout, although women are affected after menopause.

ACTION

It is best to drink 4-6 ounces of water every hour and do a fast of vegetable juice and broth for a few days. As a general preventative measure, avoid all meats, especially organ meats, shellfish, and pork, as they are high in purines which breakdown into uric acid. Also stay away from alcohol, and eat a diet low in fat and high in fiber.

KITCHEN REMEDIES

Sage–This herb eases the inflammation of gout. Make a tea and drink 1-3 cups a day.

Apple Cider Vinegar–To fight the toxins from gout, mix 1 table-spoon in a cup of hot water, sipping it 2-3 times a day.

Parsley–As a diuretic, parsley increases urination thus flushing uric acids and toxins from the body. In addition parsley has a good amount of trace minerals. Prepare a tea.

> **WARNING:** Very large doses of parsley leaf may cause nerve damage, bleeding in the gut, liver damage, and abortion.

Castor and Olive Oil–Gently rub the painful area first with castor oil, 1-3 times daily for 3 days in order to break up the urate crystals. Then rub with olive oil for three days to rebuild the system. Repeat as needed. As a preventative, this is good to do once a month.

Celery–Eat 1 or 2 stalks a day or mix a drink by blending the celery with a little water in a blender. You may add a little carrot juice for flavor. This is a great acid neutralizer and aids urine flow. Celery is high in calcium, vitamin K, and phosphorus.

Potato–Juice or blend potatoes until you have 2 ounces, then mix with 2 ounces of warm water. Drink as needed daily to fight the tox-ins in the body.

SINGLE HERBAL REMEDIES

Burdock Root–As it balances the body and increases urine flow, burdock root is excellent for gout. Make a tea.

Dandelion–Aids cleansing and rebuilding the liver, the filter and detoxifier of the body. Good amounts of trace minerals, high in cal-cium and Vitamin K. Make a tea.

Devil's Claw–Reduces joint pain and decreases uric acid levels in the blood. Foment the painful joint by applying the warm tincture or extract with a cloth or spreading the liquid with a finger directly onto the affected area. You can also drink a tea made from devil's claw.

Queen of the Meadow–This diuretic is especially good for problems concerning the kidneys and urinary tract system. In addition, Queen of the Meadow aids the aching joints of arthritis. Foment the painful joint by applying a warm tincture or extract with a cloth or spreading the liquid with a finger directly onto the affected area. reapply. In addition, make a tea.

OTHER NATURAL TREATMENTS

Fasting–It is best not to keep loading the system with more food to compound the problem. See instructions at the beginning of this book on how to fast and how to break a fast.

Soak Bath–A great relaxing tonic for the whole body. The heat helps the body eliminate toxins. While filling the tub with hot water suited to your body add single or combination of herbs desired. Use 1-2 cups of epsom salts or 1 cup of aloe vera, apple cider vinegar, or baking soda.

COMMERCIALLY PREPARED HERBAL REMEDIES

Herbs: BF&C (for bone, flesh and cartilage) capsules and ointment; Liveron (Cleans the liver and gallbladder.); Rheum-Aid Formula (for rheumatism, gout and arthritis); Kalmin (An antispasmodic extract that can be used both internally and rubbed over area.); Cal-Silica Formula (natural calcium); KB (Helps kidneys and bladder to flush uric acid that causes gout out of the system.); Ex-Stress (natural calcium and nerve support) (Nature's Way); Liquid Trace Mineral (High in minerals to balance system and can be used to soak a gouty big toe with cotton kept moist several times daily until better.); or, Calcium Citrate (Twin Lab).

Homeopathic: Raw Liver; Raw Kidney; Arthritis; Pain; or, Detoxification (Natra-Bio.); or, Arthritis Pain (Medicine from Nature).

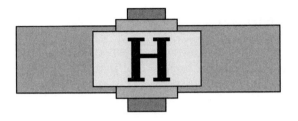

HANGOVER

If you have "partied hardy" the night before, a hangover will be evident the next morning from overindulging in alcohol. You can experience headaches, nausea, general body weakness, or dizziness and, possibly, no sympathy from anyone. Sometimes hangover symptoms may appear from an unexpected allergies or a reaction to a little alcohol in food.

> **WARNING:** If you are or have a history of addiction or alcoholism, do not use the sedative herbs, skullcap or valerian, except under the supervision of a trained herbalist. Do not use alcohol-based tinctures.

ACTION

If you are overly nervous and are drinking to try to calm the system or to build up courage, try some of these remedies instead of the debilitative alcohol. If you drink excessively or know someone who does, seek professional help. Alcoholism is a serious condition with dire physical, mental, emotional, and social consequences.

To clear alcohol out of your system, drink 4-6 ounces of water every 30 minutes for the first 2 hours then every hour after that.

133

Also, drink 2-3 ounces of water mixed with 2-3 ounces of cranberry juice 2-4 times daily for a few days. Repeat if needed. Another solution is to do an enema, particularly a coffee implant, and get plenty of sleep.

KITCHEN REMEDIES

Sage–Mix 1 teaspoon in a hot cup of water adding a pinch of cinnamon, cayenne, or ginger. Drink a cup every 1-2 hours until sober. Sage eases the queasy feeling brought on by too much alcohol.

SINGLE HERBAL REMEDIES

Skullcap–This is food for the nerves which is calming and toning. Skullcap is high in calcium, potassium, and magnesium. Take 2 capsules every hour for several hours until you are feeling better, then change to 2 capsules every 2-4 hours as needed.

Valerian–A good remedy that feeds, soothes, calms the brain and nerves. Take a little at a time, like 1-2 capsules every 2-4 hours. Or, make a tea.

White Willow Bark–This is a natural aspirin good for headaches and body aches. Make a tea.

COMMERCIALLY PREPARED HERBAL REMEDIES

Herbs: Adren-Aid Formula (Supports the adrenal glands and wakes up the system.); PC Formula (Supports the pancreas and balances the blood sugar.); Liveron (Cleanses the liver and gall bladder.); EnerGizer Formula (Picks up the system.); Liquid Trace Mineral (Take 1/2 ounce in vegetable or fruit juice about every 2-4 hours. Helps replace lost minerals due to alcohol toxicity); or, Rescue Remedy (for shock and trauma) (Bach). Also, you can try Potassium taking 1 capsule per hour for headaches and to wake up the brain and 2 capsules of Calcium Citrate (Twin Lab) or Vegetable Calcium (Schiff) every 2 to 4 hours. This also supports the nervous system.

Homeopathic: Headache & Pain; Nervousness; or, Detoxification. Take every 30 minutes for 1-3 hours, then every 1-2 hours until better. Also, try Neuralgic Pains; or, Nausea (Natra Bio.); or, Fatigue; or, Headache (Medicine from Nature).

HEADACHES

Headaches occur due to a variety of causes: muscular tension, indigestion, menstrual problems, emotional or mental stress, food toxicity or nutrient deficiency. Diseases of the head or body can also produce a headache. Some of these include infections, brain tumor, head injuries, very high blood pressure, stroke, or conditions of the ear, throat, teeth, nose, or eyes.

I have commonly noted that patients with sluggish bowels, less than 1-2 movements daily, experience many headaches. Another problem is poor posture causing a tense neck and shoulders, especially for those that type and write in a stooped position all day at work. Allergies, a stuffy room, cigarette smoke, or a foam pillow or mattress can also be the cause of the trouble.

Migraines are a very specific type of headache. They may begin with irritability, restlessness, lack of appetite, or a visual aura. Each person is different. Once the headache pain begins, it's often accompanied by nausea, vomiting, and light sensitivity. Hands and feet are often cold, and the person usually prefers to be alone in a dark room. These headaches can last for days.

ACTION

Try to determine the cause of headache: food, allergy, indigestion, menstrual period, or excessive worry and take the remedies suggested for those problems. Enemas help as well as taking potassium in place of aspirin. Alternating relaxation and rapid walks are helpful as they help to clear the mind, get the blood flowing and release inner tension. Sometimes a little food or juice helps, particularly if your blood sugar is dropping.

If you're suffering from a headache because of working too long in hot weather, then cool down immediately and drink a good bit of juice and water with a very little pinch of salt added to it. Also, try drinking an electrolyte replacement like tomato juice.

If you suffer from migraines, try eliminating foods that you may be sensitive or allergic to. There is a strong connection between migraine headaches and food sensitivity.

KITCHEN REMEDIES

Celery–Best taken as a tea, or, if you are on the run eat a couple of stalks. Dice, grate, juice, or blend about 2 ounces of celery, adding to hot water for 1 cup of tea or juice as needed. Celery is a relaxant.

Onion–Shred or grate fresh onion, then place it in a cloth bandage and tie it around the head for 20 minutes each hour. If needed, repeat with fresh onion.

Sage–This tea is very good for both headaches and mental exhaustion. Stir in 1-2 pinches of cayenne powder to the tea.

Apple Cider Vinegar–In a cool glass of water add 1/2-1 teaspoon of apple cider vinegar to stimulate the body and to get rid of the toxins. Take as needed.

Cayenne–Take 1/4 teaspoon in juice a few times daily to improve blood circulation.

Ginger–For general head pain and problems with menstrual flow, ginger tea is recommended because it stimulates circulation.

SINGLE HERBAL REMEDIES

Black Cohosh–A powerful relaxant that works well, especially for female problems and headaches in the back of the head. Make a tea.

Chamomile–Use for nerve and anxiety type of headaches. This is a relaxant that works well in the neck and shoulders area. Make a tea.

Feverfew–Works well for headaches from indigestion and migraines. Feverfew decreases the frequency and severity of migraine headaches. You must take feverfew tea for several months as a preventive measure in order to gain its effect.

Passion Flower–An overall remedy for anxiety and nerves helpful for tension headaches and relieving stress. Make a tea.

Peppermint or Spearmint–Choose this for indigestive type of headaches. Make a tea.

White Willow–A natural aspirin that relieves head and body pain. Make a tea by putting 10-20 drops of the liquid in juice or as a tea in warm water as need through the day. You can take 1-2 capsules 1-2 times a day as needed with water or juice.

OTHER NATURAL TREATMENTS

Potassium (99 milligrams)–Take 1 tablet every hour until the headache is gone. Don't take for more than eight hours.

Vitamin B Complex (50-100 milligrams)–Take 1 capsule daily to feed and calm the nervous system.

Soaking–Soak feet in hot water 1-2 minutes and then in cold for 30 seconds. This draws congested blood from the head relieving the headache pressure. If you are in hurry soak the hands instead. Sometimes an alternating hot/cold shower on the head and the shoulders helps too.

COMMERCIALLY PREPARED HERBAL REMEDIES

Herbs: Kalmin (antispasmodic) take 3-5 drops in 2-4 ounces of water every 1-2 hours. B/P Formula (Helps to relieve headaches, and the heart and circulation); CapsiCool (Cool cayenne without burning may help lack of circulation headaches); Ex-Stress (Supports and relaxes the nervous system.); Cal-Silica (Natural calcium calms system and relieves headaches.); Fem-Mend or Change-O-Life (Balances periods and estrogen imbalances.); Naturalax 1,2, or 3, or, Aloelax (These move the pressure of the toxic bowels out of the body, removing, reducing or preventing headaches.) (Nature's Way); Rescue Remedy (for shock and trauma) (Bach); Liquid Trace Mineral (Take 1/2 ounce in vegetable or fruit juice several times daily in case of electrolytes have dropped out of the system producing headaches and nausea like symptoms of heat exhaustion.

Homeopathic: Headache & Pain; Injuries; Detoxification; PMS; Menstrual; Menopause; Cold; Sinus; Aches; or, Pains (Natra-Bio.); or, Cold & Flu; Menopause; Migraine; or, Tension Headache (Medicine Nature).

HEART ATTACK

Acute heart attacks typically begin with an aching, pressure, or tightness in the chest. Often this pain travels to the back, jaw, or down the left arm. These signs are similar to those experienced with angina except they're more intense and nitroglycerin, the medication used to treat angina, does little to alleviate the attack. Shallow breathing, sweating, restlessness, paleness and a sense of impending doom may also accompany a heart attack.

> **WARNING:**   If you have any suspicion you or another person is having a heart attack, call 911. THIS IS A LIFE THREATENING SITUATION.

This is especially true if the person is unconscious or there are chest pains and an achy pain down the left arm.

ACTION

Loosen tight clothing and keep person warm if they are chilled, with feet propped up. If necessary perform cardiopulmonary resuscitation (CPR) (see Figures 35-47).

Cardiopulmonary resuscitation (CPR) involves the use of artificial ventilation (mouth-to-mouth breathing) and external heart compression (rhythmic pressure on the breastbone). These techniques must be learned through training and supervised practice. Courses are available through the American Heart Association and

American Red Cross. Incorrect application of external heart compressions may result in complications such as damage to internal organs, fracture of ribs or sternum, or separation of cartilage from ribs. (Rib fractures may occur when compressions are being correctly performed but this in not an indication to stop compression.) Application of cardiopulmonary resuscitation when not required could result in cardiac arrest, so never practice these skills on another person. When CPR is properly applied, the likelihood of complications is minimal and acceptable in comparison with the alternative—death.

CPR PROCEDURE FOR SINGLE RESCUER

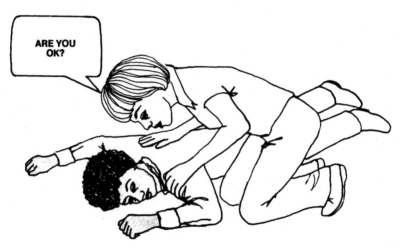

Figure 35 Recognition of Problem

The CPR procedures should be learned and practiced on a training mannequin under the guidance of a qualified instructor. The step by step procedure for cardiopulmonary resuscitation is as follows:

- Establish unresponsiveness. Gently shake the victim's shoulder and shout, "Are you OK?" The individual's response or lack of response will indicate to the rescuer if the victim is just sleeping or unconscious (Figure 35).

- Call for help. Help will be needed either to assist in performing CPR or to call for medical help.
- Position the victim. If the victim is found in a crumpled up position and/or face down, the rescuer must roll the victim over; this is done while calling for help (Figure 36).

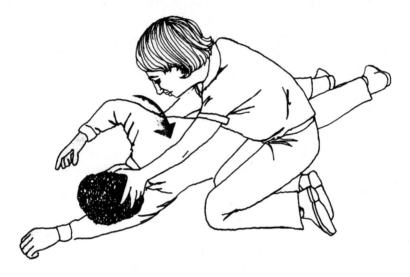

Figure 36 Turning the Victim

- When rolling the victim over, take care that broken bones are not further complicated by improper handling. Roll the victim as a unit so the head, shoulder, and torso move simultaneously with no twisting.
- Kneel beside the victim, a few inches to the side.
- The arm nearest the rescuer should be raised above the victim's head.
- The rescuer's hand closest to the victim's head should be placed on the victim's head and neck to prevent them from twisting.
- The rescuer should use the other hand to grasp under the victim's arm furthest from the rescuer. This will be the point at which the rescuer exerts the pull in rolling the body over.
- Pull carefully under the arm, and the hips and torso will follow the shoulders with minimal twisting.

- Be sure to watch the neck and keep it in line with the rest of the body.
- The victim should now be flat on his/her back.
- A-Airway. Open the airway. The most common cause of airway obstruction in an unconscious victim is the tongue.
- Use the head-tilt/chin-lift maneuver to open airway. (This maneuver is not recommended for a victim with possible neck or spinal injuries.)
- B-Breathing. Establish breathlessness. After opening the airway establish breathlessness.
- Turn your head toward the victim's feet with your cheek closed over the victim's mouth (3 to 5 seconds).
- Look for rise and fall in the victim's chest.
- Listen for air exchange at the mouth and nose.
- Feel for the flow of air (Figure 37).

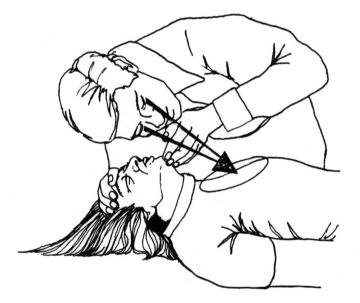

Figure 37 Establishing Breathlessness

Sometimes opening and maintaining an open airway is all that is necessary to restore breathing.

- Provide artificial ventilation.
- If the victim is not breathing give two full breaths by mouth-to-mouth, mouth-to-nose, or mouth-to-stoma ventilation (Figure 38).

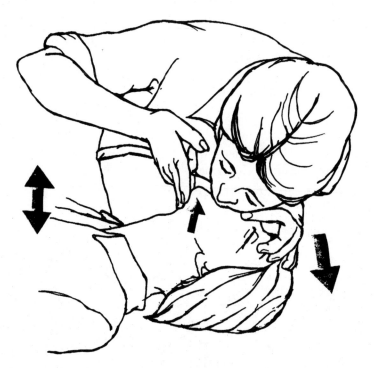

Figure 38 Two Breaths

- Allow for lung deflation between each of the two ventilations.
- C-Circulation. Check for pulse. Check the victim's pulse to determine whether external cardiac compressions are necessary.
- Maintain an open airway position by holding the forehead of the victim.

- Place your fingertips on the victim's windpipe and then slide them towards you until you reach the groove of the neck. Press gently on this area (carotid artery) (Figure 39).
- Check the victim's carotid pulse for at least five seconds but no more than ten seconds.

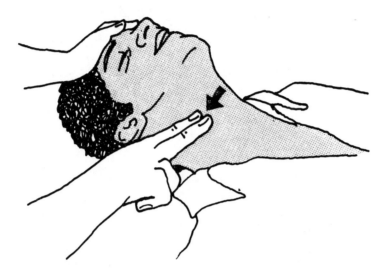

Figure 39 Checking Pulse

- If a pulse is present, continue administering artificial ventilation once every 5 seconds or 12 times a minute. If not, make arrangements to send for trained medical assistance and begin CPR.
- Perform cardiac compressions.
- Place the victim in a horizontal position on a hard, flat surface.
- Locate the bottom of the rib cage (Figures 40-41) with the index and middle fingers of your hand closest to patient's feet.
- Run your index finger up to or in the notch where the ribs meet the sternum (breastbone) (Figures 40-41).
- Place your middle finger in notch and index finger on sternum.

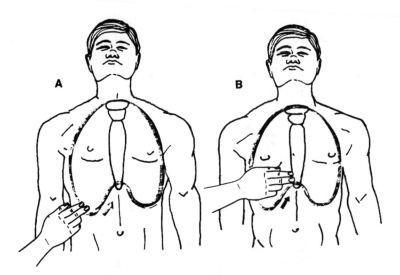

Figures 40-41 Locating the XIphoid Process

- Place the heel of the other hand on the sternum next to index finger in the notch in the rib cage (Figures 42-44).
- Place the hand used to locate the notch at the rib cage on top and parallel to the hand which is on the sternum.
- Keep the fingers off the chest, by either extending or interlocking them (Figures 42-44).

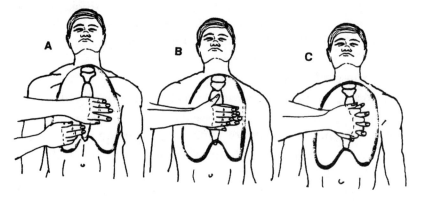

Figures 42-44 Correct Hand Position on the Sternum

- Keep the elbows in a straight and locked position.
- Position your shoulders directly over the hands so that pressure is exerted straight downward (Figure 45).

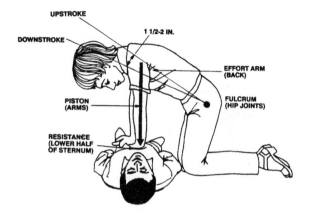

Figure 45 Exerting Pressure Downward on an Adult

- Exert enough downward pressure to depress the sternum of an adult 1 1/2 to 2 inches.
- Each compression should squeeze the heart between the sternum and spine to pump blood through the body.
- Totally release pressure in order to allow the heart to refill completely with blood.
- Keep the heel of your hand in contact with the victim's chest at all times (Figures 46-47).
- Make compressions down and up in a smooth manner.

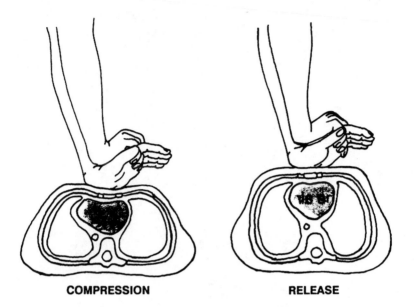

COMPRESSION   **RELEASE**

Figures 46-47 Cardiac Compression

- Perform 15 cardiac compressions at a rate of 80-100 per minute, counting "one and, two and, three and, ... fifteen."
- Use the head-tilt/chin-lift maneuver and give two full breaths (artificial ventilation).
- Repeat cycle four times (15 compressions and 2 ventilations).
- After the fourth cycle, recheck the carotid pulse in the neck for a heartbeat (5 to 10 seconds).
- If breathing and heartbeat are absent, resume CPR (15 compressions and 2 ventilations).
- Stop and check for heartbeat every few minutes thereafter.
- Never interrupt CPR for more than five seconds, except to check the carotid pulse or to move the victim.

CHILD RESUSCITATION

Some procedures and rates differ when the victim is a child. Between one and eight years of age, the victim is considered a child.

The size of the victim can also be an important factor. A very small nine-year-old victim may have to be treated as a child. Use the following procedures when giving CPR to a child:

- Establish unresponsiveness by the shake and shout method.
- Open the airway using the head-tilt/chin-lift method.
- Establish breathlessness (3 to 5 seconds).
- If the victim is not breathing, give two breaths.
- Check the carotid pulse for at least five seconds.
- Perform cardiac compressions.
- Place the victim in a horizontal position on a hard, flat surface.
- Use the index and middle fingers of your hand closest to the patient's feet to locate the bottom of the rib cage.
- Place your middle finger in notch and index finger on sternum.
- The heel of the other hand is placed on the sternum next to the index finger in the notch in the rib cage.
- The fingers must be kept off the chest by extending them.
- Elbow is kept straight by locking it.
- The shoulders of the rescuer are brought directly over the hand so that pressure downward with one hand to depress the sternum of the child 1 to 1 1/2 inches.
- Compress at a rate of 80 to 100 times per minute.
- Ventilate after every five compressions.

INFANT RESUSCITATION

If the victim is younger than one year, it is considered an infant and the following procedures apply:

- Establish unresponsiveness by the shake and shout method.
- Open the airway; take care not to overextend the neck.
- Establish breathlessness (3 to 5 seconds).
- Cover the infant's mouth and nose to get an airtight seal.
- Puff cheeks, using the air in the mouth to give two quick ventilations.

- Check the brachial pulse for five seconds.
- To locate the brachial pulse.
- Place the tips of you index and middle fingers on the inner side of the upper arm.
- Press slightly on the arm at the groove in the muscle.
- If heartbeat is absent, begin CPR at once:
- Place the index finger just under an imaginary line between the nipple of the infant's chest. Using the middle and ring fingers, compress chest 1/2 to 1 inch.
- Compress at the rate of at least 100 times per minute.
- Ventilate after every five compressions.

TRANSPORTATION OF THE VICTIM

Do not interrupt CPR for more than 5 seconds unless absolutely necessary. However, when CPR is being performed and the victim must be moved for safety or transportation reasons, do not interrupt CPR for more than 30 seconds.

When moving a victim up or down a stairway, provide victim with effective CPR before interruption Move the victim as quickly as possible and resume CPR at next level.

TERMINATION OF CPR

Under normal circumstances CPR may be terminated under one of four conditions:

- The victim is revived
- Another person trained in CPR relieves you
- The person performing CPR becomes exhausted and cannot continue
- A doctor pronounces the victim dead.

HEMORRHOIDS

Hemorrhoids, or piles, are very common. There are two types: external hemorrhoids, which occur in the anus, and internal hemorrhoids, which are situated higher. Some people can have both at the same time. Typical hemorrhoid symptoms include bright red bleeding, swelling, soreness, and burning. Itching of the anus is not usually due to hemorrhoids except when the hemorrhoids prolapse or enlarge to the point of sticking out of the anal opening. Hemorrhoids are like the varicose veins of the anus; that is, the anal veins have dilated, and in some cases a blood clot has settled there.

Besides hemorrhoids, there can be anal fissures, a more common condition than you think. Fissures are generally superficial and heal rapidly. Sometimes this groove or slit inside the anus is a painful sore or ulcerated crease which may bleed and become infected.

The events that cause varicose veins, also contribute or aggravate hemorrhoids: a genetic weakness of the veins, pregnancy, and long periods of standing or sitting. Straining too much during a bowel movement, especially from constipation, is another risk factor.

WARNING: If there is profuse bleeding, call your doctor as soon as possible. In the meantime use the suggested remedies.

ACTION

If the hemorrhoid is protruding push it back in gently. Try not to strain during bowel movements or sit too long on the toilet. Gently wipe the anal opening well after each movement, wash area gently daily. Avoid constipation by drinking more water, and eating more fiber and laxative-type foods like prunes. Use only white, unscented toilet paper.

Before applying any topical remedies, gently clean either the hemorrhoidal or anal area with natural soap and water then use natural disinfectants. Take the suggested remedies to help the bowels to move easier and. Take calcium like Ca-T (Nature's Way) or Vegetable Calcium (Schiff's) to improve vein structure.

KITCHEN REMEDIES

Aloe Vera Plant–Cut and trim the outer bark and insert the piece, like a anal suppository into the rectum for overnight healing. Repeat as needed. Aloe vera soothes and speeds healing. The soft healing plant will be absorbed and what is left will be expelled on the next bowel movement. You may also apply the squeezed gel to the anal opening.

Cayenne–If the anal opening is bleeding, cayenne helps to coagulate the blood to stop the bleeding. Put the powder on the anal opening with a moist cotton ball or cotton cloth, adding more if needed. Stop using if there is irritation.

Sage–Steep a 1/2 teaspoon of sage in a cup of hot water and apply with a cotton or leave cotton in the cheeks of the anus, repeating as needed or leave on overnight. This astringent helps heal hemorrhoids.

Garlic–Use a fresh clove of garlic, peeling it. Then moisten with vegetable oil and insert like a suppository. Leave it in overnight to act as an anti-inflammatory. Repeat as needed.

Olive, Castor, or Wheat Germ Oil–Gently apply any oil to the anal area to break up anal congestion and soothe the painful area. Take 1/2-1 teaspoon 1-2 times daily. You may follow the teaspoon of oil with a juice chaser.

Witch Hazel–Moisten a piece of cotton and tuck in the anus for about an hour or overnight to tone the anus and rectum. If the solution burns, then dilute with a little water or aloe vera plant gel. Or, add 1 quart in a tub with enough water to cover anus. Soak 10-20 minutes.

Cranberry–If bleeding, make a poultice with fresh cranberries. If you don't have fresh berries, use cranberry juice by soaking a piece of cotton and applying to the area as needed. Drinking a glass of cranberry juice also stops the bleeding.

SINGLE HERBAL REMEDIES

Pau d'Arco–Either capsules or extract can be taken internally. Extract can be applied directly to the anal opening or moisten cotton and tuck gently in the anus several times daily as needed. Great for healing sores, reducing swelling, and easing pain.

Black Walnut, or White Oak Bark–Use tincture or steep 10-20 drops in a cup of hot water, then apply directly to the anal area with cotton and repeat as needed. White oak bark is an astringent.

Bayberry–Heals and tightens. Make a tea or implant.

Burdock–Use this plant as a poultice or fomentation. It helps to heal wounds.

Marshmallow–Use this soothing remedy to ease the discomfort of hemorrhoids as a fomentation by applying warm liquid with a cloth or directly to the affected area.

Red Raspberry–This is great for healing with its iron citrate. It is good as an astringent and tonic for prolapsed hemorrhoids. Take as needed as a tea. Use as a holding injection and on cotton tucked gently into area overnight. You may lubricate the capsules with natural oil and insert as an overnight suppository.

Tormentil Root–An excellent astringent and tonic for prolapsed hemorrhoids. Take 3 ounces of extract 3 times daily or 1 ounce every 2 hours. In tincture form place 5-10 drops in 4-6 ounces of water every 1-4 hours as needed. It works well as a holding injection or implant. You may soak some cotton with the herb and place it in the anus as a suppository.

OTHER NATURAL TREATMENTS

Glycerine–One of the greatest curative, nontoxic, solvent compounds known. Acts as a nutrient and lubricant that helps heal skin diseases, wounds, and itching. Apply directly or moisten a piece of cotton that is tucked in anus overnight.

Vitamin A or E–Puncture the perle with a pin and apply to area with a finger or cotton. You can use either vitamin separately or mix them together. Speeds healing of the tissues.

COMMERCIALLY PREPARED HERBAL REMEDIES

Herbs: BF&C (Rebuilds bone, flesh and cartilage.); Red Clover Combination capsules or syrup (Purifies the blood stream.); Ex-Stress (Relaxes the nerves.); Calcium Citrate (Twin Lab); Naturalax 1,2, or 3, or, Aloelax (Nature's Way); and also take liquid trace mineral (A good healer of sores. Moisten cotton and tuck into anus overnight or during the day. It may burn if the anus is really irritated so it is best to dilute about 1/2 and 1/2 with water. Repeat as needed.).

Homeopathic: Hemorrhoids; Laxative; Varicose Veins; Pain; or, Detoxification (Natra-Bio); Constipation & Hemorrhoids; or, Indigestion & Gas (Medicine from Nature).

HICCUPS

Hiccups are the sudden rush of air caused by a spasmodic contraction of the breathing muscle, or diaphragm. This is followed by the sudden closure of the vocal chords. Hiccups can occur from eating certain foods, drinking hot or irritating liquids, from fright, nervousness, or stress. Certain conditions provoke hiccups like pregnancy, alcoholism, stomach trouble, or surgery. And sometimes, we don't know why we get hiccups.

ACTION

Try some well known hiccup treatments such as holding your breath for as long as possible, breathing through a paper bag or swallowing numerous gulps of water without taking a breath. What you are trying to do is increase the amount of carbon dioxide in your lungs to stabilize breathing. Antispasmodic or calming herbs, such as catnip, spearmint, peppermint, skullcap or valerian root teas or extracts may also help stop the hiccups and relax the diaphragm.

If hiccups are recurring, determine if the person has been eating any gassy foods like cucumbers, cabbage, or bell peppers. Chronic, severe, and breathtaking hiccups need professional medical help.

KITCHEN REMEDIES

Apple Cider Vinegar–This is a mild antispasmodic. Mix a 1/4 teaspoon or less in 4-6 ounces of warm water and sip slowly sitting upright for 30 minutes.

Cayenne–Mix a 1/4 teaspoon in 4 ounces of warm water and sip slowly for 30 minutes to work as a mild antispasmodic.

Baking Soda–Works as an antacid and relaxer for the body. Mix 1/4 teaspoon in 4 ounces of warm water and sip, taking 30 minutes sitting upright.

Ginger–A wonderful remedy that acts as an antacid, antispasmodic and helps the digestive tract in relieving gas. Make a tea with 1/4-1/2 of a teaspoon in a cup of warm or hot water and sip slowly sitting upright for 30 minutes.

Lemon or Lime–Fresh only; works as a mild antispasmodic. You can use either singularly or in combination. Mix the juice of 1/2 of the fruit in a cup of warm water. Sip slowly over 30 minutes. Dilute a little if too strong.

SINGLE HERBAL REMEDIES

Catnip–Best as a warm tea to perform as an antispasmodic and relaxer. Sip slowly, for at least 30 minutes, in seated position. Make a tea.

Chamomile or Mint Teas–To relax the nervous system, drink either one of these teas. Steep tea bag in a cup of hot water and drink slowly.

Lady's Slipper or Wild Lettuce–Either of these feeds the nerves and helps to relax the diaphragm in releasing spastic hiccups. Make a tea.

Passion Flower–This is good for nervous conditions and tones the sympathetic nervous system. Make a tea.

Valerian, Hops, or Skullcap–These herbs relax and calm the nervous system. Make a tea by putting 10-20 drops of the liquid in juice or open 1-2 capsules in a cup of hot or room temperature water, or in juice. Drink slowly, over 30 minutes, sitting upright.

Wild Yam–Best as a warm tea sipped slowly for 30 minutes to work as an antispasmodic. Relaxes muscular fiber and soothes nerves. Make a tea.

COMMERCIALLY PREPARED HERBAL REMEDIES

Herbs: Kalmin (anti-spasmodic extract); Ex-Stress (Calms the nervous system.) (Nature's Way); or, Rescue Remedy (Calms the nerves.) (Bach).

Homeopathic: Colic; Emotional; Indigestion; Nervousness; or, Pain (Natra-Bio.); or, Colic; Fatigue; or, Indigestion & Gas (Medicine from Nature).

HOARSENESS/LARYNGITIS

Hoarseness, or an unnaturally deep or harsh voice, is usually due to laryngitis or overuse of the vocal cords. An inflamed or infected larynx, or laryngitis, typically comes on suddenly. A thickly, raw throat and continuous urge to swallow characterize this condition. This infection can be caused by viruses or bacteria and often follow an upper respiratory infection or other illnesses like the measles, flu, or bronchitis.

ACTION

The best course of action is to rest the voice. Determine if you are abusing your vocal cords by singing, yelling, or talking too much, or if the condition arises from an infection. Paying attention to your diet and drinking more water are important. Also, gargle with the suggested herbs and apply some of them around your neck.

KITCHEN REMEDIES

Sage–Make a tea and use it for both a gargle and drink as needed. This is especially great for laryngitis.

Salt–Gargle with this natural disinfectant using about 6 ounces of warm or hot water, stirring in 1/4 teaspoon of salt. Gargle several times daily as needed. Spit out used water and leave in salty taste for further healing.

Fresh Garlic–Chop or mince fresh garlic (acts as a disinfectant and fights toxins), and take it with a little water. Or, you can apply it as a poultice by first rubbing some vegetable or olive oil around the neck area. You may cover this with a cloth to keep the mixture from getting on clothes. Repeat a few times during the day or overnight. You can rub a light coat of olive oil on the bottom of the feet, then rub with thick coat of fresh garlic or garlic oil. Cover feet with warm socks overnight and/or throughout the day. Repeat as needed.

Horseradish–Use the spread or grate fresh horseradish to disinfect the throat and fight the toxins. Mix with a little food and hold in the mouth several times daily. Begin by taking in small amounts and work up to a greater quantity.

Lemon–Squeeze 1/2 teaspoon of fresh lemon in a cup of hot water adding some honey, if needed, for taste. Drink throughout the day as a healing tonic and antiseptic. You can add other herbs.

SINGLE HERBAL REMEDIES

Mullein–This is great either as a tea, gargle, or fomentation for any throat and mucus problems. Take as a tea or use as a fomentation overnight or through the day.

Fenugreek and Thyme–Fenugreek works as a good cleanser and soother for the throat and lungs, while thyme thins the mucus. Drink a tea combining the herbs or take 1 teaspoon of fenugreek and 1/2 teaspoon of thyme as needed. You may also foment the neck area.

Lungwort–A good cleanser for the lungs and sinuses, and it helps to reduce mucus. Use as a tea and gargle.

Marshmallow–A great all around healing remedy that soothes the throat. Make a tea or use as gargle throughout the day.

Echinacea–Great for boosting natural immune system and cleansing general infections. You can gargle with echinacea and take as a tea. Use 10-15 drops of the extract either straight or in 4-6 ounces of water or juice as needed throughout the day.

Skullcap or Valerian Root–Either of these relaxes the nervous system. Make a tea. Gargle throughout the day or drink 2-3 times a day. Both work great in combination with other congestive relieving herbs to relax the tight vocal cords.

COMMERCIALLY PREPARED HERBAL REMEDIES

Herbs: Kalmin (anti-spasmodic); Ex-Stress (Calms the nervous system.); GL Formula (Cleanses glands and the lymph nodes.); IF Formula (Supports the immune system.); Fenu-Thyme Formula (Cleans out mucus and infections,); Breath-Aid Formula (Cleans out lung infections and congestion.); Herbal Influence Formula (for colds, flu and congestion.) (Nature's Way); or, Liquid Trace Mineral (A great healer that can be mixed with 2-3 ounces of warm water for a gargle. Take 1/2 ounce in vegetable or 1/2 diluted fruit juice and water several times daily as needed. Or, moisten cloth with mineral, wrap throat, and pin a warm cloth around the neck. Re-moisten several times throughout the day as needed.).

Homeopathic: Cough; Sinus; Earache; Fever; Laxative; Flu; Detoxification; Cold; Sore Throat; or, Cold (Natra-Bio); or, Cold & Flu; Dry Cough; or, Sinusitis (Medicine from Nature). You may also want to consult a homeopath for further help.

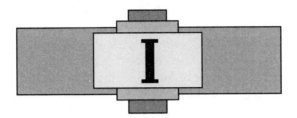

INDIGESTION

Commonly know as "heartburn," indigestion is due to stomach acid coming back up into the esophagus—the food tube that connects the mouth to the stomach. This causes a burning feeling in the chest, one which sometimes travels to the neck or even face. It usually happens after a meal, and is worse when the person lies down. How, when, and what you eat can aggravate this condition. For example overeating, eating too fast, eating the wrong combinations of foods, or eating too close to bedtime can aggravate this condition.

Other digestive problems that appear such as bloating, gas, pain, and general abdominal discomfort, particularly after eating, may occur when your stomach has too little hydrochloric acid (HCL) to breakdown food. HCL levels typically decrease as we age and in people with food allergies. Inadequate digestive enzymes may also be the cause.

> **WARNING:** If the problem continues and/or you are not sure if it is a true heart attack or pain from acute indigestion, get to a doctor or hospital soon as possible.

ACTION

Eat small, frequent meals and try to eat a better selection of foods. Eat less or no fried or greasy foods. Eat slower. If you are angry or upset, try not to eat after 7 P.M. so you can sleep better. Avoid lying down after meals, and if the heartburn affects you at night sleep with a couple of pillows.

The basic secret to quick relief from indigestion is to mix a warm 4 ounce drink with 1/4 teaspoon of either baking soda or ginger in a cup of warm water, sit in an upright position, and sip the remedy slowly for 30 minutes. Allow yourself to burp or belch, as this helps the release of trapped gas causing the indigestion.

KITCHEN REMEDIES

Baking Soda–Mix 1/4 teaspoon in 4 ounces of warm water and sip the antacid drink slowly sitting upright for 30 minutes.

> **WARNING:**   Unless your doctor supervises you, do not administer to children under 5 years old. Don't take more than 1/2 tsp. 8 times a day if you're under 60 years old or 1/2 tsp. 4 times a day if you're over 60 in a 24-hour period. Don't use baking soda if you're on a sodium-restricted diet.

Ginger–Mince or grate enough fresh ginger to make 1/4 teaspoon, then add to a cup of warm water. This acts as a carminative, thus promoting gastric secretions and is good for gas. Sip for half an hour while sitting upright. Can also use ginger root or the dried herb from the health food store.

Sage–This herb eases stomach upset. Drink the tea slowly for at least 30 minutes, sitting upright.

Peppermint/Spearmint–Most mint teas will work; however, spearmint or peppermint are great for indigestion as they both relax the stomach, promote digestive secretions and bile flow and are antispasmodics. Drink 2-3 times a day, especially after meals.

Cloves–Place a few cloves in a cup of hot water to settle a queasy stomach and steep for a few minutes and sip. Can also use clove oil.

Blessed Thistle or Cornflower–Mix 1/2 teaspoon in 6 ounces of hot water for a natural antispasmodic. Let the cornflower settle or strain and sip slowly.

Potato–Blend 2 ounces of fresh potato in a blender to make an antacid and antispasmodic. Then mix with 2 ounces of water and drink slowly. Or, slowly chew a large piece of raw potato.

Soft Drink–If nothing else is on hand, as usually is the case, slowly sip 4-6 ounces of carbonated soda or water to burp up gas. This trick worked on an elderly couple traveling across the Arizona desert. They called me long distance from a little store in the middle of nowhere. The wife thought she was having a heart attack but it sounded more like a severe gas attack after eating at a greasy spoon restaurant about an hour earlier. There were no herbs, alkaseltzer, or baking soda available so I had her slowly sip, for at least 30 minutes, the cola drink while sitting upright. In about 5 minutes she belched several times and felt much better.

Garlic Oil–Either uses 5-10 drops or 1/2 capsule in a cup of warm water for a mild antispasmodic. Can also use fresh garlic.

> **WARNING:**   Garlic may cause indigestion in some people.

Parsley–Works as a mild antacid and antispasmodic. Use 1 capsule in 6 ounces of water.

> **WARNING:**   Very large doses of parsley leaf may cause nerve damage, bleeding in the gut, liver damage, and abortion.

SINGLE HERBAL REMEDIES

Chamomile or Fennel–These are great for in relieving gas. Make a tea.

> **WARNING:**   Large amounts of fennel can disturb the nervous system.

Skullcap or Valerian Root–Either of these fights toxins and relaxes the nerves. Good for a nervous stomach. Make a tea.

Wild Yam–A great remedy to assist in the relief of gas and stomach pains due to its antispasmodic action. Make a tea.

COMMERCIALLY PREPARED HERBAL REMEDIES

Herbs: Kalmin (antispasmodic) or Kol-X (For stomach gas and relieves indigestion and colic. Try 5-8 drops in warm water or warm juice. Sip for 30 minutes while sitting upright to aid burping and belching. Repeat as needed.); Ex-Stress capsules or extract (Calms digestive and nervous system.); Naturalax 2 or, Aloelax (Nature's Way); or, Yeast Fighters (Releases gases and yeast.) (Twin Lab). For chronic indigestion problems try various digestive enzymes with meals, such as, Schiff's Emzamall or Digest Aid by Dr. Jensen.

Homeopathic: Indigestion; Laxative; Colic; Emotional; or, Candida Yeast (Natra-Bio); or, Colic; or, Indigestion & Gas (Medicine from Nature).

INSECT REPELLENT

We all like to spend some time out in the wonders of nature, yet those pesky fleas, flies, mosquitoes, gnats, and other various insects can hamper a good hike, picnic, hunting or fishing trip, or camping expedition. In order not to get bitten or stung, natural insect repellents are provided. (See "Bites/Stings" for treating stings and bites.)

ACTION

For the best results, apply the repellent before going out. You can fill a small plant sprayer or atomizer with the concoction to spray on the skin, or fill a bottle to rub it on. Be sure to take extra with you.

KITCHEN REMEDIES

Apple Cider Vinegar–Apply directly onto the skin or mix with a little vegetable oil. Also, it is good to add 1 teaspoon 1-2 times daily in the diet.

Olive and/or Wheat Germ Oil–Apply lightly over the skin. Blend in a ratio of 1 to 1 or use singularly. To dilute the oils, you may add some vegetable oil.

Witch Hazel–Apply directly onto the skin or use a spray bottle to disperse.

Garlic or Onion–After finely chopping, dicing, mincing, or grating the fresh garlic and/or onion, mix with some wheat germ or vegetable oil and apply. If you are using the powdered garlic or onion, it needs to be soaked in one of the oils for a few days before use. You can add crushed or powdered basil leaves to this mixture.

Vanilla–Rubbing vanilla on your skin before going out helps ward off the bugs (and it smells nice too.)

SINGLE HERBAL REMEDIES

Repellent Mixture–Mix equal parts of: rosemary, basil, wormwood, and rue plus 1 teaspoon of apple cider vinegar and a little olive oil to help it stick to the skin. Then, place the mixture in a glass bottle and set it in the sun inside for 2 days. Shake well before using. Rub or spray on the skin. Also, this is a great healer for bites and stings.

Brewer's Yeast–Mix 1 tablespoon in food, in a hot water drink or soup. Protects from the inside out. Take 1-3 tablets 1-2 times a day. Do **not** use this remedy if you have any kind of yeast or fungal infection, or are allergic to yeast.

Eucalyptus Oil–Mix 10-20 drops with a little water or vegetable oil and rub or spray over the skin.

Garlic Oil and/or Goldenseal–Mix up a 1 to 1 blend of olive oil, garlic oil and/or goldenseal. Rub the concoction directly on the exposed skin.

Penny Royal–Rub or spray onto exposed skin.

OTHER NATURAL TREATMENTS

Thiamine Tablets (B-1)–This vitamin helps to produce a natural insecticide manufactured by the body. Take 2 tablets (50 mg) 1-2 times daily before going into the woods or being outside.

Vitamin E (200-400 IU)–Puncture the perle, squeezing out the oil onto the skin and spread. You also can mix the vitamin E with a little vegetable oil. To help your pets, lightly rub or spray some vitamin E into the fur, but keep it away from the paws and the face.

COMMERCIALLY PREPARED HERBAL REMEDIES

Herbs: Rub any of these on the skin. BF&C, Comfrey, Chickweed ointment; Kalmin (An antispasmodic for bites and to repel bugs.); AKN Skincare Formula (Cleanses the skin and wards off biting insects); Mix Echinacea Combination with other herbs, like Black Walnut Hull extract, Pau d'Arco Bark, or garlic oil, directly on the skin as natural insect repellent and good to apply to bites. It can be taken internally as well.); or, Liquid Trace Mineral (Good for bites and stings on the body).

Homeopathic: Insect Bites, or, Detoxification (Rub either on the skin or combine them to avoid bites.) (Natra-Bio); SssstingStop (Soothing repellent and bug gel.). Also, see various natural bug repellent sprays and gels available at your local health store. Besides taking the homeopathic, you may apply it directly to the bites.

INSOMNIA

If it is frequently difficult for you to go to sleep or return to sleep after being awakened, then you are dealing with insomnia. Many of us suffer from sleeplessness at one time or another. In fact, at least one-third of Americans complain of insomnia each year. The causes vary from too much worrying, or planning going on in your mind, being exhausted, eating too much before bed, or indigestion. Alcohol, caffeine, drugs, and some medications may interfere with sleep as well. If your problem is chronic and the following suggestions don't help, consider visiting with your doctor. Insomnia can be a symptom of depression (see "Depression") or anxiety (see "Anxiety/Phobias"). More serious sleep disorders such as sleep apnea or narcolepsy may also be responsible.

ACTION

If your mind is busy with all sorts of notions, try deep breathing and slowly exhaling to relax, or, counting backwards from 100. Eliminate alcohol and caffeine from your diet. Avoid taking stimulating herbs like ephedra before bedtime. Exercise during the day (but not too close to bedtime) will also help you relax and sleep. In addition, refer to the recommended remedies below for help.

KITCHEN REMEDIES

Herbal Teas–Sage, catnip, peppermint, or spearmint teas should be drunk about 1 hour before bedtime to relax and induce sleep. Some grocery stores and health food stores have these teas in bag form; however, if you only have loose herbs then make an infusion.

Milk–Drink a warm cup of goat, whey, or cow's milk before going to bed. Milk is a source of tryptophan which produces a calming chemical in the body to help you sleep.

SINGLE HERBAL REMEDIES

Blue Vervain–This is a natural tranquilizer. Make a tea and drink about an hour before going to sleep.

Catnip, Chamomile, or Valerian Root Extracts–These are all great relaxers. Make a tea. Drink 1 hour before bedtime to relax.

Lady's Slipper or Skullcap–Both are natural tranquilizers that work particularly well for an exhausted nervous system. Make a tea. Drink 2-3 times a day.

Passion Flower–Great for the hyperactive child or if you are experiencing restlessness, exhaustion or agitation. Make a tea. Drink 2-3 times a day.

OTHER NATURAL TREATMENTS

Enema–Mix 1 teaspoon of baking soda or the juice of 1/2 of a **fresh** lemon with seeds strained, into a bag of warm distilled or spring water and use as an enema. An enema releases toxic fecal matter from the bowels to help you relax and sleep better.

Exercise–Try walking, running, biking, or bouncing on a rebounder to burn off extra energy, aggravations, or whatever is bothering you. It is best to this several hours before bedtime or early in the day.

Music–Listen to relaxing music or subliminal sound tapes like the rain or the ocean to help you drift off into sleep.

Shuffle Walk–Shuffle in your bare feet through the grass for about 10 minutes in the early evening, and, if needed again, before going to bed as a way to relax. This activity discharges the built up negative and excessive static electrical charges that have accumulated throughout the day.

COMMERCIALLY PREPARED HERBAL REMEDIES

Herbs: Kalmin (anti-spasmodic); Silent Night (Aids sleep.); Ex-Stress (Relaxes the nervous system.) (Nature's Way); drink Sleepy Time tea; or, Rescue Remedy (for shock and trauma) (Bach). You can also take 2-3 tablets of Calcium Citrate (Twin Lab) before going to bed.

Homeopathic: Insomnia; Nervousness; Exhaustion; or, Emotional (Natra Bio.); or, Colic; Teething; Fatigue; or, Insomnia (Medicine from Nature).

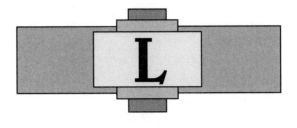

LICE

Lice are a parasitic infection. Depending on the variety, the louse can be found on the head, the body, or in the groin area. Pubic lice are often referred to as "crabs." Both children and adults may be infected.

The head louse is transmitted by personal contact or by using infected objects like combs, brushes, headgear, or sleeping on an infested pillow. Although associated with dirty, cramped conditions, head lice are very common among school-aged children especially where coats and hats are hung in an open cloak room.

Crabs or pubic lice are passed through sexual contact. Body lice are difficult to find on a person's body since these parasites live in clothing such as underwear. Thus, wearing infested clothing can cause an infection.

Intense itching is very characteristic of lice. Sometimes a secondary infection can develop from excessive scratching. The body louse may also carry typhys, trench fever and relapsing fever. To discover the lice, use a magnifying glass and inspect the head hair, groin or underclothing. The adult louse is often hard to see, but its nits or eggs can be easily identified. The difficult-to-remove nits look like pussy-willow buds on hair, close to the scalp or skin.

WARNING: Lice are very difficult to get rid of. While they're
usually not dangerous, they are bothersome. Even after taking
all precautions and treating the infected person, the lice may
return if you don't kill or remove all nits. You won't know if you
are successful for at least a month.

ACTION

Clean and disinfect the affected body area with a mixture of straight
apple cider vinegar, garlic oil, and black walnut husk extract. Use a
fine tooth comb and vinegar rinse and remove all the nits from anyone who has head or pubic lice. Soak all hair brushes, combs and hair
accessories in a lice shampoo or the above solution.

All clothes, bed linens, towels—anything in which the infected
person has come in contact with—needs to be washed with a good
biodegradable soap along with 1-2 cups of apple cider vinegar added
to each load of clothes, daily. Items that can't be washed, may be
placed in large, plastic bags and kept there for a week or in the freez-
er for three days. Vacuum all carpets, upholstery and mattresses, and
dispose of the vacuum bag in the outside garbage.

Dr. John Christopher, in his book, *Childhood Diseases* recom-
mends spraying the room 1-2 times a day with a concoction made of
six parts chaparral, three parts black walnut bark and one part
lobelia or Kalmin, plus, add few drops of lavender oil or oil of mint
for fragrance to each pint of spring water. You may also use this mixture in the laundry. Then try a recommended remedy.

Inspect all household members for lice. Inform anyone that has
been in contact with the infected person that they should be exam-
ined for lice. This is especially crucial for school age children. Some
schools forbid children with lice from attending classes until they
have been treated. If you have crabs, inform your sexual partner(s)
and urge them to seek treatment.

KITCHEN REMEDIES

Aloe Vera–Apply after or between other treatments for healing the
bites. Take a leaf and slice open to apply the gel inside.

Apple Cider Vinegar–Apply directly to the area of soreness by rubbing the apple cider vinegar or put some into a spray bottle. Take 1/2 teaspoon in water or an alkaline juice like apple juice 2-3 times daily. Also, try a soak bath (see below).

Garlic or Onion–Grate or chop fresh garlic, or an onion to help as antiseptics, then mix with vegetable oil or apple cider vinegar and apply. You may also add a little in some juice or food 3-4 times daily. Massage garlic oil into the infested area leaving in 1-2 hours, then wash hair or leave it in overnight with shower cap on.

SINGLE HERBAL REMEDIES

Black Walnut Husk Extract or Pau d'Arco–A great parasite cleanser is black walnut husk extract. Use to wash clothing and bed sheets (see Action section). Take as a tea and rub through the hair and over the skin several times daily. Use black walnut husk extract in a soak bath to rid the body of the lice. While filling the tub with hot water suited to your body add a single or combination of the herbs desired. Tinctured or liquid teas are very good here. If you are not able to find black walnut husk extract, then use the infection fighter Pau d'arco as a substitute.

Chaparral–This is good for various skin parasites, especially scabies. Since the tea is very bitter, it is best to take the capsules or tincture in juice or other minty teas. Use in a soak bath to rid the body of the lice.

Echinacea–Take 1-3 capsules or 10-15 extract drops in water or juice 2-3 times daily as needed. Echinacea is a great infection fighter.

Thyme–Thyme oil is best for external use. Mix 4 drops of oil with 4 ounces of olive oil or aloe vera gel. You may also add in 10 drops of black walnut tincture to mixture. Use in a soak bath to rid the body of the lice. If you feel you need to take thyme internally, take 30-50 drops of tincture or 2 capsules 2-3 times daily for adults and use 5-10 drops 1-2 times daily for children.

OTHER NATURAL TREATMENTS

Soak Bath–A great relaxing tonic for the whole body. While filling the tub with warm water suited to your body add 1/2 cup of apple cider vinegar.

COMMERCIALLY PREPARED HERBAL REMEDIES

Herbs: Red Clover Combination (blood stream purifier); Myrrh-Golden Seal Plus (A hair, skin and blood purifier.); Para-X (Cleans various parasites.); Naturalax 1,2, or 3, or, Aloelax (Nature's Way); Rescue Remedy (For shock and trauma because some people can get very upset about having lice.) (Bach); or, liquid trace mineral (To delouse add 1-2 cups of the mineral to a soak bath or apply full strength directly to the infected area.).

Homeopathic: Insect Bites; Detoxification; or, Hair & Scalp (Natra Bio). Take and apply to area. Various companies have natural insect repellents that are available in your health store.

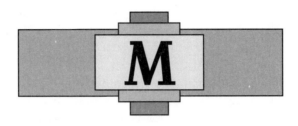

MENSTRUAL PROBLEMS

Menstrual problems range from a suppressed or absent menstrual period (amenorrhea), painful periods or cramps (dysmenorrhea) to excessive bleeding (menorrhagia) and irregular bleeding or spotting between periods.

Dysmenorrhea, or menstrual cramps, is by far the most common menstrual problem affecting about half of all premenopausal women. Symptoms may include lower abdominal cramping, backache, nausea, and vomiting. Some of the symptoms of premenstrual syndrome (PMS), like bloating, irritability and weight gain, can also accompany menstrual cramps. This condition can be totally debilitating or an annoying discomfort. A hormone-like substance in the body, called prostaglandins, are thought to be in too high when cramps occur. High levels of estrogen, a female hormone, also make dysmenorrhea worse.

Amenorrhea, or no menstrual period, can be due to a variety of things. One fairly common cause is crash dieting and anorexia nervosa. Obesity and emotional distress can also block menstruation. If any of the many hormones that trigger menstruation are imbalanced, flow can stop or decrease. Serious illness and some drugs like barbiturates, opiates, and steroids can also stop a period. There are times when menstruation ceases because of normal, physiological events: pregnancy, menopause, breastfeeding.

Menorrhagia is what doctors call excessive menstrual bleeding. The problem with this condition is how to evaluate what is considered excessive. Usually the doctor must estimate from her patient's story and the number of tampons or pads she uses how much menstrual blood flows each month. Besides hormonal factors or serious illness, increased menstrual bleeding can happen when the woman has uterine fibroids, polyps, or cancer, an ectopic pregnancy (where the fertilized egg is implanted somewhere other than the womb), from an IUD, when taking anti-clotting drugs or when the woman is deficient in vitamin K. (See "Bleeding".)

Finally, spotting or bleeding at times other than your menstrual period is called metrorrhagia. Irregular bleeding results from a variety of causes including forgotten tampons, infections, excessive douching or trauma, endometriosis, cancer, and hormonal imbalances. It's important that you figure out if the bleeding is actually coming from the vagina, or is it from the urinary tract or bowel. Some women experience spotting when they ovulate. If a young girl, too young to menstruate, is bleeding vaginally this may be due to trauma or sexual abuse.

> **WARNING:** If you experience sudden vaginal bleeding, particularly with pain, call your doctor immediately. If there's excessive vaginal hemorrhaging soon after childbirth this may be due to a retained placenta, call 911 (See "Bleeding."). If you're pregnant, call your doctor anytime you bleed vaginally. If you have a young daughter who is bleeding vaginally, contact the proper authorities if you suspect sexual abuse or rape.

ACTION

A healthy lifestyle and diet of course help many health problems including those related to menstruation. Exercise at least three times a week by walking, biking, playing tennis, or any other sport, especially benefits menstrual cramps. Keep the bowels and kidneys open by drinking more water and try the suggested remedies.

KITCHEN REMEDIES

Sage–Add to the tea 1/2 pinch of cayenne pepper to fight the toxins that may be causing the problem.

Beet Juice–This is great especially for the suppressed period. Beets are food for the liver, an organ which converts estrogen to its less active form. Treating the liver is an excellent way to treat menstrual problems in general. Mix 1 ounce of beet juice in 2 ounces of apple or carrot juice. Drink 2-3 times daily. Beet juice also improves circulation builds the blood and regulates the menstrual cycle.

Carrot Juice–Drink 4-6 ounces 1-2 times daily.

Witch Hazel–The astringent quality of this plant makes it appropriate for excessive periods. Take 15-60 drops or 2-3 capsules 2-3 times daily.

HERBAL REMEDIES

Black Cohosh, Cramp Bark, or Chamomile–Any of these remedies help to relieve cramps, painful and excessive periods, and hard-to-start periods. For a singular remedy tea put 10-20 drops of the liquid in juice or open 1-2 capsules in a cup of hot or room temperature water, or in juice. For a combination tea mix 5 drops or 1/2 capsule of each remedy, either two or all three in juice or a cup of hot water. Drink tea 2-3 times a day.

Catnip–Helps suppressed menstruation and the diarrhea, nausea, and cramps of dysmenorrhea. Make a tea.

Dong Quai or Siberian Ginseng–Dong quai is a strong but gentle, natural regulators of an imbalanced menstrual cycle. The estrogen-like substances it contains has made it a popular traditional remedy for most menstrual complaints. Siberian ginseng, on the other hand, build stamina both physical and mental. Make a tea with either herb.

False Unicorn Root–False unicorn root is a great male/female hormone balancer that assists irregular and painful periods. This herb works well with cramp bark. Make a tea.

Peppermint–Performs great for cramps and menstrual related headaches. Make a tea.

Red Raspberry–Use this remedy for nausea, cramps, and painful and excessive bleeding as a tea, vaginal implant, or douche. Make a tea. You can mix red raspberry with equal parts of goldenseal in a douche for menstrual cramps.

WARNING: Do not use goldenseal if you are pregnant or have hypoglycemia.

OTHER NATURAL TREATMENTS

Foot Bath–Soak feet in hot water for 10-15 minutes with 1/2 cup of epsom salt. The hot water draws blood from the internal female organs to the feet, pulling out heavy impurities. Works great for painful and suppressed periods.

Soak Bath–A great relaxing tonic for the whole body. Soak 1-2 times during the anticipated week of your menstrual period, especially if you are having a suppressed period. While filling the tub with hot water add 1-2 cups of epsom salts.

COMMERCIALLY PREPARED HERBAL REMEDIES

Herbs: Ex-Stress (Calms the nervous system.); Fem-Mend Formula or Change-O-Life (female support); Calcium Citrate (Twin Lab); Rescue Remedy (for shock and trauma) (Bach); Paulsfre (Michael's); or, Ladies Only (period regulator) (Crystal Springs).

Homeopathic: Menstrual; Emotional; Pain; or Raw Female (Natra Bio); or Vaginitis (Medicine from Nature).

MISCARRIAGE, THREATENED

Miscarriage or the threat of it can be a frightening event. Signs of a threatened miscarriage are vaginal bleeding and/or cramping of the womb during the first half of a pregnancy. While we often don't know what causes this, a malformed fetus is often the reason especially if the miscarriage occurs in the first trimester. Infections like German measles or herpes and chronic illness such as diabetes can also induce a miscarriage. There are times, however, when a woman's womb or other reproductive organs have difficulty holding a baby. While this chapter in no way is meant to replace the important services of your physician during a threatened miscarriage, I do offer some natural remedies that you can try along with your doctor's treatments.

> **WARNING:** If you begin bleeding or having unusual cramps while pregnant, call your doctor immediately. Lie down and prop your feet up, keep warm and calm.

Remember the cardinal rule of pregnancy: don't take any medication, natural or otherwise, unless you absolutely need to. For safest results, consult with a practitioner trained in natural medicine before taking any herbs.

PREGNANCY NOTE

You should absolutely avoid these herbs while pregnant: barberry, bloodroot, calamus, cascara sagrada, cayenne, celandine, ephedra, fennel, flaxseed, goldenseal, juniper, lavender, licorice, male fern, mayapple, mistletoe, passion flower, pennyroyal, periwinkle, poke root, rhubarb, sage, tansy, thuja, thyme, wild cherry, wormwood, yarrow.

These herbs should be used with caution and only under the guidance of a trained herbalist while pregnant: alfalfa, angelica, burdock, calendula, chamomile (German), dong quai, fennugreek, feverfew, ginger, gotu kola, horehound, hyssop, lemon balm, motherwort, nettles, peppermint, plantain, milk thistle, St. John's wort, and uva ursi.

KITCHEN REMEDIES

Olive or Wheat Germ Oil–Apply either warm oil over the abdomen, keeping warm and quiet with the feet either level or slightly elevated.

SINGLE HERBAL REMEDIES

False Unicorn Root–This remedy, from the Native Americans, is a great tonic and reproductive system strengthener. It helps balance and tone all troubles with the womb. This herb can be taken freely throughout pregnancy particularly for threatened miscarriage. Use as a tea.

WARNING: Excessive amounts may cause nausea and vomiting.

Cramp Bark–An antispasmodic herb that relaxes the uterus and calms the nerves, helping to prevent a miscarriage. Make a tea and drink three times per day.

Wild Yam–Excellent in relieving cramps due to a miscarriage. Make a tea and take as needed.

Valerian Root–Performs as a great muscle and nerve relaxer. Works well with cramp bark. Make a tea and drink 2-3 times a day.

White Willow Bark–A natural headache and pain reliever that is safe for both mother and fetus. Make a tea.

COMMERCIALLY PREPARED HERBAL REMEDIES

Herbs: Red Raspberry (Great for nausea and strengthening the female system.); Kalmin (anti-spasmodic); Ex-Stress Formula (Calms the nervous system.)

Homeopathic: Injuries; Emotional; Nervousness; Pain; or, Headaches (Natra-Bio); or, Fatigue; or, Headache (Medicine from Nature).

MOTION SICKNESS

Traveling in a car, airplane, train, or a boat sometimes produces dizziness, overall body weakness, nausea, vomiting, feelings of panic, cold sweating, sleepiness, and an upset nervous system. Overstimulation, through movement, of the balancing organs in the inner ear cause motion sickness. However, other factors can aggravate this situation. Emotional reactions to feeling homesick, being somewhere you would rather not be or going where you do not want to go play a role. Watching a moving horizon, sitting in a stuffy vehicle filled with smoke, fumes or carbon monoxide and a low blood sugar also contribute to motion sickness.

ACTION

The best treatment for motion sickness is prevention. Improve diet by not overeating or drinking alcohol, and change lifestyle by doing some exercises and not staying up too late. When traveling do try not to lay down, read, or watch the horizon rolling by, or look out of a car window. You might want to move to a steadier seat in an airplane such as a seat over the wings, or on a boat move to some place midship. Most of the suggested remedies can be taken during the trip, so ask an attendant for hot water to mix up your selected remedy or carry a thermos with the premixed remedy in it. Also, try taking some herbs for the pancreas and low blood sugar listed on page 176.

KITCHEN REMEDIES

Baking Soda–This is an easy way to make antacid. Mix 1/4 teaspoon in 4 ounces of warm water and sip slowly over 30 minutes while traveling.

WARNING: Unless your doctor supervises you, do not administer to children under 5 years old. Don't take more than 1/2 tsp. 8 times a day if you're under 60 years old or 1/2 tsp. 4 times a day if your over 60 in a 24-hour period. Don't take this maximum dose for more than 2 weeks. Don't use baking soda if you're on a sodium-restricted diet.

Ginger–Helps to overcome nausea from the motion of the vehicle. Make a tea from ginger powder or the fresh root. You can also use ginger capsules or extract from the health food store.

Cloves–Carry some with you and suck or chew on them like gum. Cloves settle your stomach and help prevent nausea and vomiting. Drink a tea of fresh cloves before you leave and while you are on the trip. Ask for a cup of hot water when you are in a restaurant and on an airplane, train, or boat to steep cloves in and drink it.

Sage–Brew tea before trip and take some to drink during trip to help as a soothing tonic and to settle an upset stomach. If you are on a trip, sage extract or capsules from the health food store may be easier to carry and use than home brewed tea. Take 2 capsules or put 10-20 drops of the extract or open 2 capsules into a cup of hot water. Take 2-3 times a day while on your trip.

Peppermint or Spearmint–You may find already prepared tea bags in the grocery or health food store. Some restaurants also offer these teas. If you can only find the loose leaves, then prepare tea following the directions at the front of the book. Both of these remedies calm the nervous system, allay nausea, and are antispasmodic.

Honey or Raisins–Taking a little honey or eating raisins during the trip keeps your blood sugar up.

SINGLE HERBAL REMEDIES

Red Rasberry or Ginger—Either of these herbs will settle the stomach down in a few minutes. You can repeat each hour as needed.

COMMERCIALLY PREPARED HERBAL REMEDIES

Herbs: PC Formula (Balances the pancreas and blood sugar.); Motion Mate (Helps counter motion and/or a pancreas drop in blood sugar.); Adren-Aid (Balances adrenal glands and regulates the heart.); Ex-Stress (Calms the nervous system.); Liveron (Supports and cleanses the liver and gall bladder.) (Nature's Way); or, Rescue Remedy (for shock and trauma) (Bach).

Homeopathic: Nausea; Emotional; Detoxification; Headache & Pain; Laxative; or, Exhaustion (Natra-Bio). It is best to take these homeopathic remedies a few days before a trip when possible or at least 30 minutes before leaving and carry them with you. Some health stores carry other help for motion sickness problems.

MUMPS

The first signs of mumps are chills, headache, loss of appetite, malaise, and a mild fever. About a day later, inflammation and swelling of the neck and salivary glands occur along with a rise in fever. The swelling makes it painful to swallow. Although this seldom occurs, the testicles may become inflamed and swell in young men. Mumps last a few days to a week.

ACTION

Get plenty of bed rest and either do an enema or take herbs to help the bowels move to break the fever and reduce painful swelling due to toxins. Food intake should include natural vegetable broth, baked potato (no skin), and various juices. Drink 6 ounces of water for adults, and 3 ounces for children, every 1-2 hours. And take a suggested remedy.

KITCHEN REMEDIES

Apple Cider Vinegar–Acts as a great antiviral. Drink a cup of hot water mixed with 1/4 teaspoon apple cider vinegar and cover up. Repeat 2-3 times a day.

Cayenne Pepper–In a cup of hot water or hot apple juice add 1/4 teaspoon of cayenne pepper. This is also a great additive to other herbs listed below. Cayenne is an antiseptic that helps cleanse the blood of toxins and stimulates blood circulation.

Sage–Drink the prepared tea to fight the infection while soothing the body. You may add a 1/4 teaspoon of ginger or cayenne to speed healing.

Garlic or Onion–Grate or chop fresh garlic or onion and mix in a hot tea and drink. Or, add to warm vegetable oil and apply to swollen neck.

Ginger–Make a tea using only 1/4 teaspoon of ginger. You can also add a 1/4 teaspoon of sage. In addition, make a poultice and apply it around the neck.

SINGLE HERBAL REMEDIES

With any of the following herbal remedies you may foment the mumps as well as take internally. For fomentation apply the warm oil or liquid with a cloth onto the affected area. Keep the cloth moist by re-soaking the cloth in the warm solution several times a day. To keep the cloth moist in between the applications, wrap and pin a dry towel or cloth over the wet one. You can also use a heating pad over the dry towel or cloth to keep the fomented cloth warm.

Red Raspberry–This is great for various viral childhood infections. Take either in capsule form or as a tea.

Mullein–Great for any glandular swellings as it breaks up the congestion and fights the infection. Also, add 1/4 teaspoon of valerian root extract to your mullein tea to relax the body. Can drink as a tea and apply as fomentation around the neck as needed.

Myrrh–This is a great anti-infection fighter. Take as a tea.

Fenugreek–Cleans excess mucus out of the respiratory system. Make a tea or use as a gargle for sore throats.

Boneset–Excellent for all viral type of infections, and, if there is fever, aching, and chills. Make a tea.

Echinacea–A good blood purifier and infection fighter that gives immune system support. Make a tea with only echinacea or add it to any of the above listed herbs to help boost the immune system.

Cornflower (Yellow best)–Used by the Native Americans of the Plains for infectious diseases. Mix 1/2 teaspoon of cornflower in 6-8 ounces of hot water and take 2-3 times daily.

OTHER NATURAL TREATMENTS

Enema–Mix the juice of 1/2 a **fresh** lemon with seeds strained, into a bag of warm distilled or spring water. Use this mixture as an enema.

COMMERCIALLY PREPARED HERBAL REMEDIES

Herbs: GL Formula (Cleanses the glands.); Fenu-Thyme Formula (Clears the glands and congestion.); Ex-Stress (Calms the nervous system.); or, Liquid Trace Minerals (A great healer of aches and infections. Apply directly on the mumps or soak a cloth or cotton ball with the mineral and apply. Also, take about 1/2 ounce in 4-6 ounces of vegetable or fruit juice several times daily as needed.).

Homeopathic: Fever; Detoxification; Sore Throat; Nausea; Earache; Headache & Pain; Flu; Fever; Pain; or, Raw Thymus (Natra-Bio); or, Earache; or, Headache (Medicine from Nature).

MUSCLE CRAMPS

Muscle cramps can be due to a variety of causes. Cramps in the leg muscles can become tight, spastic, painful, and sore. Often this condition is caused by either the lack of or poor absorption of calcium, potassium or magnesium.

ACTION

Improve your diet by eating more fresh vegetables, fruit, and whole grains. Eating foods with too many preservatives, or, too much refined sugar in them, causes the calcium to be leeched out of the body. Also, reduce your intake of coffee and alcohol.

KITCHEN REMEDIES

Spearmint, Peppermint, or Catnip Tea–Any of these herbal teas act as an antispasmodic and relax the nerves. You can purchase tea bags at a grocery or health food store. Or, if you have loose herbs prepare you own tea.

Castor Oil–Warm the oil and rub it into the muscles to relax and feed them.

Olive Oil–This soothes and rebuilds the muscle. For severe cramping take 1 teaspoon every 2 hours with a juice chaser. Apply oil either warm or at room temperature gently over the tender muscle. Repeat every 1-2 hours as needed. In addition, you may apply a hot, wet towel or cover the sore, oiled muscle with a towel and place a heating pad turned on to a low setting over the sore muscle.

Wheat Germ Oil–Feeds, tones and strengthens muscles. Wheat germ oil provides natural vitamin D and E. Take 1-2 teaspoons 1-2 times daily with juice or on salads. You can also rub on the oil and lay in the morning or late afternoon sun for 5 minutes and increase up the time to about 10-20 minutes a day. Sunlight is an important source of vitamin D.

SINGLE HERBAL REMEDIES

Black Cohosh–Works as an antispasmodic for the muscles and is a sedative. Make a tea and drink 2-3 times a day.

Chamomile–Relaxes and helps sore muscles. Drink as a tea and use as a fomentation.

Cramp Bark–This is especially good for muscular tension and spasms. Drink as a tea and use as a fomentation.

Liniment Formula–Mix 1-2 teaspoons of myrrh tincture, 1 teaspoon of goldenseal and 1/2 teaspoon of cayenne in 1 quart of rubbing alcohol (70 percent solution). You can also mix 2 ounces or 2 capsules of powdered myrrh, 1 ounce or 1 capsule of powdered goldenseal and 1/2 ounce or 1/2 capsule of cayenne pepper in a quart of alcohol. Also, you may add 1 teaspoon or 2 capsules of prickly ash, a circulatory stimulant, for chronic problems. Mix well and let it stand for seven days, shaking well daily. On the eighth day strain and throw out any residue. Great relief for various aches and pains.

Marshmallow–Soothes and relaxes the muscles. Drink as a tea and use as a fomentation.

Passion Flower–This sedative herb is especially good for twitching muscles. It eases muscle spasms and may be used with other herbs. Apply as a fomentation and drink as a tea.

Vervain, Valerian, or Skullcap–Any of these are great strong sedatives and relievers of muscle pain and spasms. Vervain and skullcap are also nerve tonics which feed and tone the nervous system. Each of these plants can be taken as a tea or used as a fomentation for cramped muscles.

OTHER NATURAL TREATMENTS

Soak Bath–A great relaxing tonic for the sore leg muscles and the whole body. While filling the tub with hot water add single or combination of herbs desired, such as catnip, peppermint, or spearmint. Or use 1-2 cups of epsom salts or 1 cup of aloe vera, apple cider vinegar, or baking soda.

COMMERCIALLY PREPARED HERBAL REMEDIES

Herbs: Kalmin (anti-spasmodic); Cal-Silica Formula (natural calcium); Ex-Stress Formula (Calms the nervous system); capsules or

ointment (bone, flesh and cartilage rebuilder) (Nature's Way);
Vegetable Calcium (Schiff) or Calcium Citrate (tissue and nerve
support) (Twin Lab.); liquid trace mineral (Good for cramps and an
electrolyte balancer. Take 1/2 ounce of the mineral in 4-6 ounces of
vegetable or fruit juice 2-3 times daily as needed.); or, Rescue
Remedy (for shock,trauma, and accidents) (Bach).

Homeopathic: Exhaustion.; Injuries; or, Aches & Pains (Natra-Bio);
Fatigue; or, Injury & Backache (Medicine from Nature); or,
Calcarea Carbonica, 3-6X potency (Suggest 1-2 tablets 2-3 times
daily with other calcium additives. This enhances calcium absorption.).

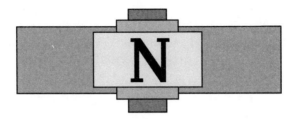

NAUSEA AND VOMITING

Generally nausea or vomiting can be caused by a variety reasons from food that has spoiled, overeating, greasy foods, drinking too much alcohol, food poisoning, and morning sickness. Taking vitamins, minerals, and herbs on an empty stomach sometimes causes nausea so take supplements with a little bit of food. Long trips also make some people nauseated (see "Motion Sickness"). If your nausea persists, it may indicate an inner ear problem. See your doctor if this is the case, particularly if it's accompanied by dizziness.

> **WARNING:** If you are nauseated and vomiting due to pregnancy, consult with your physician before taking anything, including herbs. See "Pregnancy Note" under the "Miscarriage, Threatened" section.

KITCHEN REMEDIES

Basil or Sage–Both of these herbs are carminatives, meaning they help the body release gas. They also ease the discomfort of nausea and vomiting. Make a tea using 1 teaspoon of either herb or combine 1/2 teaspoon of each. You can also add a pinch of cinnamon.

Baking Soda–Mix 1/4-1/2 teaspoon in 4-6 ounces of warm water for a natural antacid. Sip slowly for 30 minutes. Use this alkaline substance sparingly.

Apple Cider Vinegar–Take 1/2-1 teaspoon with a little honey. This is particularly good for morning sickness. Sip slowly before sitting up. Mixing the apple cider vinegar water with your saliva balances your pH to aid in digestion. When pregnant taking this along with a plain cracker before sitting up will help absorb excess bile.

Cayenne, Cinnamon, Cloves, or Ginger–Any of these are great as a preventiveness for vomiting. Take as teas.

Lemon–Use fresh lemons only. Squeeze the juice of 1/2 of a lemon in a cup of warm water. A little honey to sweeten is optional.

Coffee–This is an old Italian remedy that helps relieve nausea, gas, indigestion, or vomiting if no other remedy is available. It's particularly effective after eating rich foods or overindulging. Drink 1/2-1 cup of black coffee with no sugar or cream. Sip slowly in an upright position for 30 minutes.

Carbonated drinks–When nothing else is available, any carbonated drink such as seltzer or soda pop helps an upset stomach by causing you to belch. Slowly sip four to six ounces while sitting upright for 30 minutes.

Foods to Eat–If you have morning sickness during pregnancy, before getting up in the morning eat a small portion of apples, raw potatoes, crackers, melba or plain toast. These foods will help stabilize your blood sugar.

SINGLE HERBAL REMEDIES

Red Raspberry–This is great for most nausea, food poisoning, and morning sickness. Make a tea.

Aloe Vera–Mix 1-2 teaspoons of the liquid juice in a little water or other juices to soothe the stomach lining. Sip slowly.

WARNING: Don't drink more than a quart of aloe per day.

Peppermint or Spearmint Oil–Make a strong antispasmodic tea for vomiting. Make a tea by putting 30-50 drops of the oil in a cup of hot or room temperature water. Drink 2-3 times a day.

> **WARNING:**   Be cautious about taking peppermint when you're pregnant.

Valerian Root–Use this antispasmodic for vomiting and morning sickness as it calms the nervous system. Make a tea by putting 15-30 drops of the liquid in a cup of hot water. You may add 1/4 teaspoon of valerian root to a cup of catnip tea. Drink 2-3 times a day.

Wild Yam–Performs as an antispasmodic for both morning sickness and vomiting. Make a tea by putting 10-30 drops of the liquid in a cup of hot or room temperature water. Drink as needed throughout the day.

COMMERCIALLY PREPARED HERBAL REMEDIES

Herbs: Kalmin (antispasmodic); Motion Mate (for motion type nausea) (Nature's Way); or, Rescue Remedy (if feeling emotional) (Bach), 2 capsules of LG (Nature's Way) 3 times daily.

Homeopathic: Nausea; Detoxification; Nervousness; Fever; Emotional; or, Colic (Natra-Bio); or, Headache (Medicine from Nature).

NIGHTMARES

Many times nightmares are due to eating or drinking too much close to bedtime. Fatigue and fevers can also spark bad dreams.

ACTION

Change your liquid intake habits by cutting out all refined or processed sugar drinks, like sodas. Skip the late night heavy snack and try some herbal teas, especially before bedtime and try a suggested remedy. Also, see "Insomnia" and "Anxiety/Phobias."

KITCHEN REMEDIES

Chamomile or Sage–Either herb calms the nervous system and works as an antispasmodic for twitching muscles during sleep. You can purchase prepared tea bags at your grocery or health food store, or if you have the herb loose, make a tea. Drink a cup of tea before bedtime.

Thyme–Take 1 hour before bedtime to improve sluggish digestion. You can also drink this tea 2-3 times daily.

Marjoram–Take this as a tea about one hour before bedtime to calm the nerves.

SINGLE HERBAL REMEDIES

Catnip–Take catnip as a tea one hour before going to bed as this is great for bad nightmares. It relaxes the body's system.

Peppermint or Spearmint Oil–Either of these herbs calms the nerves and the stomach. Make a tea by putting 5-8 drops of either oil in a cup of warm juice or hot water. Drink as needed before bedtime.

Skullcap or Valerian Root–Each of these calms the nervous system. Make a tea and drink before bedtime.

OTHER NATURAL TREATMENTS

Sleep Position–If you lie on your back while you sleep, try sleeping on your side. Also, change the bed position in the room. For example, place the head of your bed toward the north or opposite direction if the bed is already there. You might change the side of the bed you sleep on too. A 42 year old man came to us having terrible nightmares. I asked if he slept on his back or his side, the wife said on his back. When changing positions from his back to his side he had no more nightmares.

COMMERCIALLY PREPARED HERBAL REMEDIES

Herbs: Cal-Silica Formula (natural calcium); Kalmin (anti-spasmodic); Ex-Stress Formula (Calms the nervous system); Silent Night (sleep aid) (Nature's Way); Calcium Citrate (Twin Lab) or Vegetable Calcium (Schiff); Rescue Remedy (for shock and trauma) (Bach); or, Calm (Hyland).

Homeopathic: Insomnia; Indigestion; Injuries; Headache & Pain; Menopause; Laxative; Exhaustion; Emotional; or, Detoxification (Natra-Bio); Fatigue; or, Indigestion & Gas (Medicine from Nature); or, Calcarea Carbonica (Enhances calcium absorption and may relieve bad dreams.). Also contact a homeopath for Sulph 200X for a chronic problem with nightmares if the other herbs suggested are not working.

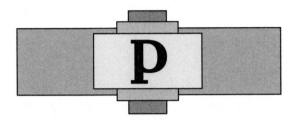

POISONS

Poisons come in many forms—solid, gas, or liquid—and from many sources: pesticides, household cleaning products, poisonous plants, food poisoning (see "Food Poisoning"), drugs, fumes like carbon monoxide from cars and chemicals. Medications and street drugs can also poison a person, either by an accidental overdose or an intentional suicidal gesture.

The symptoms of poisoning vary greatly depending on the source, amount ingested, the time since ingestion, and the size, age, sex and health of the person. They include salivation, thirst, vomiting, diarrhea, fever, abdominal pains, cramps, feeble pulse, dilated pupils, excessive urination, difficulty in breathing, spinal paralysis, convulsions, and even death. You will notice that many of these symptoms, such as diarrhea and vomiting, are ways in which the body tries to rid itself of the poisons.

Poisoning among children usually happens when a common household product is ingested because of lack of supervision. It's very important to keep all potential poisons high and out of reach of small ones. Alcohol can also cloud thinking and cause accidental poisoning among adults. Alcohol taken with otherwise safe doses of medication, like barbiturates, can be lethal.

WARNING: In all cases of poisoning, first call your local Poison Control Center, hospital or 911 for instructions and possible transport. This is especially important if the person is having difficulty breathing.

ACTION

The best way to treat poisoning is through prevention. Keep potentially poisonous substances out of reach of small children. Watch your children carefully. Teach your children not to put anything like garden plants in their mouth. Don't handle poisons while intoxicated.

If poisoning has already occurred, follow these first aid steps. If two people are present, have one treat the victim and the other call for help.

FIRST AID TREATMENT

1) Dilute the ingested poison by having the victim drink water or milk. Do this only if the person is conscious. Stop if he becomes nauseated.

2) If the person is unconscious and/or not breathing, do CPR (see "Heart Attack"). If person is choking, see section on "Choking".

3) If person vomits, save a sample for the hospital or doctor. If the person is unconscious while vomiting, turn him on his side so he won't choke. DO NOT INDUCE VOMITING IN SOMEONE UNCONSCIOUS OR HAVING CONVULSIONS.

4) Only use the following treatments on the advice of a physician, hospital, or Poison Control Center. The exception to this rule is if you're unable to immediately contact or travel to a medical facility, as in camping. Then induce vomiting as described below only if an overdose of drugs have been taken, and if you're absolutely sure the person hasn't ingested a petroleum product, or strong acid or alkali. Then go to a medical facility as soon as possible.

5) If someone is having convulsions, see section on "Convulsions."

You can induce vomiting with:

a) Syrup of Ipecac: 1 tablespoon for children, 2 tablespoons for adults.

b) A more natural emetic is mixing 10-20 drops each of: Irish moss, prickly ash bark, and cayenne pepper in 1 quart of distilled or mineral water with a dissolved ounce of sodium sulfate (optional).

c) Can also induce vomiting by sticking your finger down your throat.

You can absorb toxins with:

a) Activated charcoal–1 or 2 tablespoons mixed in a glass of water.

You can give a laxative:

a) Epsom salts–1 tablespoon mixed in a liquid for adults; half this amount for children.

CALLING FOR HELP AND GATHERING INFORMATION

1) Call Poison Control. Give them the age of the victim, type and amount of poison (if known - see #2), first aid being used, if person has vomited, and your location and how long it'll take to get to the nearest hospital or doctor. Tell them if you need an ambulance or police escort.

2) Try to determine the source of the poisoning, such as spoiled food, inhaled or ingested poisonous sprays or insecticides, or drinking an acidic juice in pottery cups that may have arsenic or lead residues that react to juice.

3) Save the container and/or label of the poison if known. If not, a sample of vomit will help the doctor identify the poison.

DO NOT try to neutralize the poison with lemon juice or vinegar. This may harm the victim more.

DO NOT give the person any type of oils, like olive or castor. They cause harm if inhaled into the lungs.

DO NOT follow antidote information on the bottle of the poison. Sometimes these are incorrect. Only administer antidotes on the advice of a physician, Poison Control Center or hospital.

CORROSIVE AGENTS, STRONG ACIDS AND ALKALIS, PETROLEUM PRODUCTS You can tell when corrosive poisons have been swallowed by burns around the mouth and on the lips. Strong acids include such substances as liquid toilet bowl cleaner. A strong alkali is oven cleaner or drain cleaner. Petroleum products, such as gasoline and kerosene, can be identified by a strong gas smell emanates from the person.

DO NOT give water or milk to someone who has swallowed these products. It may induce vomiting, and if this occurs the poison may cause more chemical burns in the person's mouth and esophagus.

Your doctor may advice you to induce vomiting in a case of petroleum poisoning. However, only do so with his supervision.

Otherwise follow the general directions for poison first aid.

PROSTATE, ENLARGED

The prostate is a small, walnut shaped gland that is part of the male genital system. This gland's job is to secrete a milky substance that neutralizes the semen and vagina so sperm can effectively fertilize an egg. One of the most common conditions affecting this organ is called benign prostatic hyperplasia or BPH. This means the prostate is unusually large. Symptoms, which strike half of men between 40 and 59 years of age, include increased urination, an urge to urinate without results, frequent nighttime urination, and a weak urine stream that stops and starts. These symptoms result from the enlarged prostate pushing on the urinary tract.

If chills, high fever, low back pain, and aching joints accompany these symptoms in a man, he may have prostatitis. This is a more serious problem and often requires hospitalization and a doctor's care. Bladder infections may follow if the prostatitis isn't treated right away. Sometimes chronic prostatitis develops as part of BPH.

> **WARNING:** Check with your doctor if you have signs of prostatitis: fevers, chills, low back pain, aching muscles, and urination problems.

ACTION

Check for occupational hazards, such as sitting or driving for too long of a time. Sit on a better seat or use a donut hole cushion in the office or car to take the strain and pressure off of the prostate. Do more walking or any other kind of light, moving exercise, drink more water, and take a soak bath at least 2 times a week. Eliminate or reduce your coffee and alcohol intake. In addition to using the suggested remedies, check with your doctor.

Men over the age of 40 should have their physicians check their prostates every year not only for BPH but prostate cancer as well.

KITCHEN REMEDIES

Sage–Works as an antiseptic, blood cleanser, and overall body tonic. When you make this tea you may add a pinch of ginger and cayenne.

Cranberry Juice–Mix 2 ounces of cranberry juice in 2 ounces of water drinking 2-3 times daily. This juice acts as an antiseptic tonic that cleanses the urinary tract and kidneys.

Parsley–Helps resistances to infections and diseases, acts as a cleanser, and is high in iron and minerals. Make a tea by putting 1 teaspoon in a cup of hot water or steep a handful of fresh parsley for 5 minutes. Let the tea cool and drink 1-3 cups daily for a few days.

> **WARNING:** Very large doses of parsley leaf may cause nerve damage, bleeding in the gut, liver damage, and abortion.

Corn Silk–A great cleanser of the urinary tract, bladder, and prostate. If you have fresh corn with silk tops, cut a good handful steeping 5 minutes in a quart of water. Drink 4 ounces every 1-2 hours. Otherwise obtain tea from a health store. A farmer called complaining of a swollen prostate and infrequent urination. I had him steep some of his fresh corn silk. After three days his swelling was down and urination was back to normal.

Castor and Olive Oil–Apply castor oil to swollen or painful area to help break up congestion or stagnation of the prostate. Do this for 3 nights, then use olive oil for the next 3 nights. Olive oil assists in feeding the prostate.

SINGLE HERBAL REMEDIES

Saw Palmetto–This plant, a native of Florida, is a popular herbal remedy for benign prostatic hyperplasia. Take as a tea.

Panax Ginseng–This ginseng is used a lot in Oriental Medicine for a variety of problems. Ginseng increases the male hormone, testosterone and helps shrink an enlarged prostate. Take as a tea or capsules.

Burdock Root or Queen of the Meadow–Both of these diuretics work great for an enlarged prostate. Make a tea and drink 2-3 times a day.

Buchu–Good for genital-urinary tract problems as it works as a tonic and cleanser. Make a tea and drink 2-3 times a day.

OTHER NATURAL TREATMENTS

Soak Bath–A great relaxing tonic for the whole body and good treatment for cleansing the body of toxins. Use 1-2 cups of Epsom salt or 1 cup of aloe vera, apple cider vinegar, or baking soda.

Zinc (50 milligrams)–This mineral is needed for good prostate function. For a chronic prostate problem, take 1 tablet daily. Reduce in about 3 weeks to 1 tablet every two days. Don't take high doses of zinc for more than two months as it interferes with copper absorption.

COMMERCIALLY PREPARED HERBAL REMEDIES

Herbs: Kalmin (antispasmodic); Red Clover Combination (Purifies the blood stream.); Cal-Silica Formula (natural calcium); Ex-Stress Formula (Calms the nervous system.); PR Formula (Cleanses the prostate.); Naturalax 1, 2, or 3, or, Aloelax (Nature's Way); liquid trace minerals (Take 1/2 ounce in 4-6 ounces of vegetable or fruit juice several times daily. Also use 1 cup of the mineral in a 30 minute soak bath for prostate.); Vegetable Calcium (Schiff), or, Calcium Citrate (Twin Lab).

Homeopathic: Prostate; Raw Male; Detoxification; Injury; Laxative; Emotional; or, Pain (Natura-Bio); or, Fatigue; or, Injury & Backache. (Medicine from Nature).

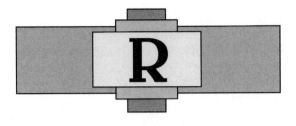

RASHES

Skin rashes are exceedingly difficult to diagnosis, even for physicians. They can be caused by so many different things such as psoriasis, poison ivy or oak, impetigo (caused by staphylococcus or streptococcus), scabies (an irritating skin mite), allergies, or a nervous state. Rash symptoms range from skin irritation that itch, redness to inflamed pustules.

One of the most common rashes are hives which are a reddish, itchy rash that can resemble a patch of insect bites. Hives are typically an allergic reaction to drugs, bites or stings, or foods. Sometimes hives can occur from an emotional problem, such as, held in resentment, fear, anger, or worry. The following remedies are general suggestions to help temporarily cope with skin rashes until a definitive diagnosis can be made. A naturopathic physician can offer you appropriate natural cures for skin ailments.

ACTION

You may be able to determine the cause of the rash yourself. Take a look at the soap you use, laundry detergent, fabrics you wear, jewelry you wear, or anything else that comes in contact with your skin. Any of these things may cause an irritation or rash called contact dermititis. Sometimes food allergies cause rashes too. If you suspect you're sensitive to a particular food, try eliminating it from your diet for a week or two and see what happens.

If you've been unusually tense recently, try some stress releasing techniques (see "Anxiety..."). Have you been hiking or in the woods lately? The rash may be from poison ivy or insect bites. (See "Bites/Stings").

Wash the rash with a natural soap and water. Then carefully apply a natural disinfectant and one of the below remedies.

KITCHEN REMEDIES

Sage–You may use this remedy in several different ways to treat rashes. Sage helps to fight the toxins in the body and soothes the nerves. Drink as a tea, apply as a fomentation, or use in a soak bath (see below). Mix the sage leaves or powder with a little water or vegetable oil to make a paste and apply to the worse areas of the rash.

Meat Tenderizer–This is a great remedy because the papain from the green papaya fruit enzyme neutralizes the poisons of most rashes. Mix the amount needed to cover the rash with a little water or vegetable oil to make paste and apply.

Baking Soda–Relieves the itching. Mix the amount needed to cover the rash with a little warm water to make paste and apply as needed.

Aloe Vera–Good for all types of rashes, burns, irritations, bites, stings, and poison ivy or oak because it not only soothes the skin but also fights infection that may be causing the rash. The gel from inside the leaf is the best to use as it adheres better to the skin. Mix some gel with water and drink.

WARNING: Do **not** take internally when pregnant.

Buttermilk–Spread the milk directly on the rash as needed to work as toxin fighter and to soothe the skin.

Apple Cider Vinegar–This is good for poison ivy or oak to soothe the skin and fight the toxins. Take a 1/4 teaspoon in a cup of warm water 3-4 times daily. Also apply directly to the area with a clean cloth as needed.

Avocado Oil–Use a little at a time and massage into the skin well, especially good for psoriasis. Acts as an antiseptic and soothes the skin rash.

Oatmeal–Cook 2 cups in 2 quarts of water for about 15 minutes in a cloth bag to neutralize the toxins in the rash. Pull the bag out, cool to warm and squeeze gently over area. If you have no cloth make a bag out of thin towel, cook, strain and apply.

Wheat Germ Oil–This is a tonic for the skin and relieves the itching. Take 1 teaspoon 2 times daily and apply lightly to the rash.

Witch Hazel–Apply directly to the rash with a clean cotton cloth, especially good for poison ivy or oak and bites that works as an astringent and speeds healing.

Celery–Settles the nervous system and works well for hives. Eat fresh stalks, or blend with a little water to make a juice, 4-6 ounces, and drink. Or, steep 1/2 teaspoon of celery seeds in a cup of hot water. Strain and drink. A great tea for quick relief.

SINGLE HERBAL REMEDIES

Plantain–One of the best for relieving rashes, especially poison ivy or oak because it astringent quality draws out toxins and as a demulcent it's soothing to painful and itchy skin. Make a tea and drink 2-3 times a day. You may also use 1 tablespoon or 2 cups of strong plantain tea as a soak bath.

Black Walnut–This is particularly good for rashes from poison ivy or oak, fungal infections, eczema, and herpes as it acts as an antiseptic and soothes the skin. If you are breast feeding do not take in large amounts, such as 20 drops and up or 2 capsules over 4 times daily for many weeks, as it may stop lactation.

Burdock Root–Works well for rashes and bites that are caused by a systemic imbalance. Particularly effective for dry, scaly conditions such as psoriasis, eczema, and dandruff as well as poison ivy or oak. Also heals wounds and ulcers when applied externally. It is an antiseptic and it tones the skin. Take 30-50 drops straight, 2-3 capsules or put drops into a hot cup of water to make a tea 3-4 times daily as need. Apply fomentation too.

Chickweed–Works great for rashes that itch and are irritating such psoriasis and ecemza. Make a tea by putting 1 tablespoon of the liquid in a cup of hot or room temperature water, or in juice. Drink 2-3 times a day. You may also use 1-2 cups of chickweed tea as a soak bath.

Red Clover–A great blood cleanser that is particularly good for psoriasis and other chronic skin problems. Very safe for eczema in children. Make a tea.

Taheebo Extract–This is a good antibiotic and antifungal for rashes, especially psoriasis. Drink as a tea and foment.

Oregon Grape–A great blood cleanser for various skin problems that works especially well for staphylococcus. Very good for chronic skin rashes such as eczema, psoriasis and acne. Take as a tea and apply as a fomentation.

WARNING: Do not use during pregnancy.

OTHER NATURAL TREATMENTS

Vitamin Complex of A (10,000 IU), D (200-400 IU), or, E (200-400 IU)–Take 1 tablet daily and puncture a perle, squeezing the contents directly onto the rash and spread to soothe the skin and fight the toxins.

Soak Bath–A great relaxing tonic for the whole body. The heat opens the pores in the skin and aids in elimination of any toxins. Soothes rashes. While filling the tub with hot water suited to your body add 2 tablespoons of sage, oat straw or a combination of herbs as desired. Use steeped bulk tea, 1-2 cups of the prepared tea, or place some bulk herbs in a clean sock tied at the end. Place this in the running water and leave in during the bath to use as an herbal wash cloth in lieu of soap. Use 1-2 cups of Epsom salt or 1 cup of aloe vera, apple cider vinegar, or baking soda.

COMMERCIALLY PREPARED HERBAL REMEDIES

Herbs: Kalmin (anti-spasmodic); BF&C (Rebuilds bone, flesh and cartilage.); Red Clover Combination capsules or syrup (Take and apply to area for various rashes.); AKN Skin Care Formula; Liveron (Cleanses the liver and gall bladder); Ex-Stress Formula (Calms nerve endings.); or, Liquid Trace Mineral (This is good for healing various rashes. Apply directly to the rash and take 1/2 ounce in 4-6 ounces of vegetable or fruit juice several times daily. You can also use 1 cup in a 30-minute soak bath.).

Homeopathic: Laxative; Nervousness; Poison Oak & Ivy; Detoxification; or, Candida Yeast (Natra-Bio).

SCIATICA

Sciatica begins as low back and hip pain that can be mild or extreme. Very often it is accompanied by a neuralgic or shooting pain that runs through one or both buttocks and down the leg. This pain follows the sciatic nerve that runs from the low back down to the back of the thigh. A variety of things can cause sciatica ranging from degenerative joint disease in the spinal bones to a slipped or ruptured disc. Fractures, infections, or tumors in the back may also cause sciatica. When someone carries a lot of weight on their belly due to obesity or pregnancy, the back can suffer.

Not surprisingly, this condition becomes more common the older you get. By the time people reach 60, about half of them have experienced sciatica. The situations that aggravate sciatica and weaken your back are occupational stress from your job or in the home, or the way you stand, lifting, sleeping, and inadequate nutrients.

Also, sciatica could be due to toxic poisons and sluggish bowels, especially the sigmoid colon and cecum which puts pressure against the lower back, leg nerves, and blood vessels, sometimes causing numbness or tingling sensations.

ACTION

Improve the diet by eating more fiber, drinking more water, taking enemas and herbs to clean the bowels. Improve occupational standing, lifting, or sleeping habits. Try chiropractic adjustments or a naturopathic physician who works the neuro-lymphatic pressure points in the low back, especially with reactive muscles. Visit with an osteopathic physician or naturopathic doctor who is familiar with soft tissue techniques that can be used on the back. Traction may be useful as well as therapeutic massage. Make sure your practitioner gives you appropriate exercises to strengthen and stretch your back. This is important not only for treatment, but prevention as well. Have your doctor show you the exercise, watch you perform the exercise, and then watch you again in a week or two to make you're doing them properly. These need to be done daily. In addition to physical treatment, apply the suggested remedies.

KITCHEN REMEDIES

Apple Cider Vinegar–Bathe feet in hot, but comfortable apple cider vinegar. For faster relief, place one foot in hot vinegar and rub bottom of other foot with a little olive oil, then with liquid garlic oil. Or, place olive oiled foot into pan of freshly chopped garlic. This really gets the circulation moving and relieves the pain. Take 1 tablespoon of apple cider vinegar in about 1 teaspoon of honey 2-3 times daily. Can also use as fomentation to sore area by applying warm vinegar with a cloth or directly to the affected area.

Wheat Germ Oil–To feed and relax the muscles, gently massage the warm oil onto the lower back and buttocks.

Cayenne Pepper–Take 1/4 teaspoon in tea or juice. Foment by applying the warm tea of cayenne with a cloth or directly to the sore area to relax the nerves. Keep moist by adding the liquid to the cloth or redampen cloth by immersion and reapply.

Garlic–Apply as a poultice. Before using the poultice put vegetable or olive oil over the area first. You may use a warm heating pad over the low back and buttocks. The heat allows the warm oil and garlic to relax and gently stimulate the taunt nerves bringing relief. For overnight help, first lightly rub some olive onto the feet, then place chopped garlic in a pair of old socks securely on the feet to keep the them in place.

HERBAL REMEDIES

Burdock Root–A great cleansing herb that aloe works as an antiseptic. Take as a tea and apply as a fomentation. Before fomenting rub either warm olive or wheat germ oil to the sore muscles. Then apply the warm tea with a cloth or directly to the affected area.

Chaparral–Detoxifies the bowels, cleanses the system, and acts as a rebuilding herb. Relieves the pain, specifically, of sciatica. Works particularly well with equal parts of burdock root. Take and foment. Make a tea and drink 2-3 times a day.

Garlic Oil–This is a great cleanser and antiseptic that relieves bowel gas and toxins that place internal pressure against the sciatic nerve. Take as a tea and apply the oil to area after first applying olive or vegetable oil to protect area. You may cover the oiled area with towel and apply heat. In addition, you can mix any of the following oils together for massaging. Make a tea by putting 5-8 drops of the oil in a cup of hot or room temperature water. Drink 2-3 times a day.

Peppermint Oil–Works as an antiseptic and antispasmodic that is great for stomach and bowel pain. Mix 5-8 drops of oil in a cup of hot water, herbal tea, or juice and drink 2-3 times daily. Additionally, mix 1 tablespoon of peppermint oil equally with olive or vegetable oil, increase for amount needed to use or store if necessary. Warm before applying to sore, painful areas several times daily as needed. You may mix any of the listed oils together for massaging.

Sassafras or Rosemary Oil–Sassafras purifies the blood and neutralizes many poisons in your system. Mix equal parts of either or both oils with warm olive or vegetable oil and massage into sore areas. If necessary, you may apply heat with a hot towel or heating pad. Also, you can take either oil, 3-5 drops, or 10-20 drops of the liquid extract, in hot herbal tea or juice. Drink 2-3 times daily as needed.

Thyme Oil–An ancient remedy that is both antiseptic and anaesthetic (numbing) to the skin and sensory nerves. Use small doses internally for effectiveness. Take as a tea and mix as a liniment. Make a tea by putting 3-5 drops of the oil in a cup of hot or room temperature water, or in juice. Drink 2-3 times a day. To make the liniment mix for *children* combine 2 parts of olive oil to 1 part thyme oil; for *adults* mix 1 part olive oil to 1 part thyme.

OTHER NATURAL TREATMENTS

Soak Bath–Use 1 tablespoon of ginger and/or 1-2 cups of apple cider vinegar as great relaxing tonics for the whole body. Also, you can use 1-2 cups of Epsom salts or 1 cup of aloe vera or baking soda.

COMMERCIALLY PREPARED HERBAL REMEDIES

Herbs: Cal-Silica Formula (natural calcium); Naturalax 2, or, Aloelax; Ex-Stress Formula (Calms the nervous system.); BF&C (Rebuilds bone, flesh and cartilage) capsules and ointment; Kalmin (anti-spasmodic) (Nature's Way); Vegetable Calcium (Schiff), or, Calcium Citrate (Twin Lab); or, Rescue Remedy (for shock and trauma) (Bach).

Homeopathic: Neuralgic Pain; Laxative; Exhaustion; Emotional; Pain; or, Detoxification (Natra-Bio.); Injury & Backache.(Nature's Way); or, Sciatica (Biological Homeopathic Industries).

SINUSITIS

Sinusitis is inflammation in the sinuses either from an infection or allergy. This condition may be long term or acute. Symptoms include sinus drainage, runny nose, congestion, sinus headaches, toothaches, sneezing, difficulty breathing, fevers, and chills. Viral infections in the upper respiratory system, colds, and flus can lead to sinusitis.

ACTION

Take an enema, improve diet by eating more vegetables, fruits, fiber, and drink more water. Since allergies can cause sinusitis, especially long-term cases, experiment by eliminating suspected foods or staying away from probable causes like cats and dogs. You can also enlist your doctor's help in pinpointing the exact allergens. Occasionally yeast infections may aggravate chronic sinusitis. If your sinusitis follows a cold or flu, see "Cold/Flu" section for more suggestions.

KITCHEN REMEDIES

Sage–Brew the tea and use for a drink, nose drops, and a gargle. You may also add 1/2 teaspoon of ginger and/or a pinch of cinnamon or cayenne to a cup of sage tea. For nose drops, clean an old nose dropper and bottle or buy an empty one from a druggist and put some tea into the bottle for use. Store the nose drops in a cool place out of the sunlight and heat.

Salt–Mix 1/4 teaspoon of salt in a cup of warm water and place a few drops in nose. If it burns the mucus membranes, then it's too strong and needs to be diluted with more warm water until the burning stops. To store the nose drops solution, clean an old nose dropper and bottle or buy an empty one from a druggist. Also, great as a gargle for the sore throat from dripping sinuses.

Garlic or Onion–Grate or chop either one or both of these fresh vegetables. Mix either individually or together in a little apple cider vinegar and add some honey for taste. Take a little at a time, working up to 1/2-1 teaspoon 3-4 times daily.

Horseradish–Works as a decongestant. Grate a little fresh horseradish into juice or apple cider vinegar and hold in the mouth for a few minutes. Also, mix in the food. Start with small amounts and work up to 1/2-1 teaspoon 3-4 times daily. Great to use on a regular basis for sinus problems.

SINGLE HERBAL REMEDIES

Liniment–This is great to apply around the sinus area, neck and chest as decongestant. Combine 1 teaspoon of tincture or 2 ounces of powdered myrrh with 1/2 teaspoon goldenseal tincture or 1 ounce of powder, and 1/4 teaspoon of cayenne tincture or 1/2 ounce of powder in 1 quart of rubbing alcohol (70 percent solution). Let it stand several days and shaking well daily. Strain into separate bottle, then use as needed.

Mullein or Myrrh–Either is powerful as an antiseptic for the mucus membranes. Take as a tea, gargle, and put a few drops in nose for sinuses infections. Make a tea. For nose drops, clean an old nose dropper and bottle or buy an empty one from a druggist and put some tea into the bottle for use. Store the nose drops in a cool place out of the sunlight and heat. Use the nose drops or gargle as needed.

Peppermint–Put 5-10 drops of oil in hot water, and with a towel over the head breathe in the vapor. A side benefit of this steam treatment is that it's a great facial. Make a tea and drink 2-3 times a day.

Eucalyptus Oil–This relieves the stuffed up sinuses. Put a few drops of the oil in the nose. Also, put 5-10 into a bowl or pot of hot water, draped with a towel over the container and head, hold the head over the hot steam and inhale deeply so that it goes up the nose.

Fennel–Helps relieve the sinuses. Take the tea as needed and place a few drops of the tea in the nose. Make a tea and drink 2-3 times a day. **Caution:** Large amounts can disturb the nervous system.

Boneset–This is great for deep chills and achy bones that can sometimes accompany sinus problems. Also relaxes mucus membranes and clears congestion. Make a tea and drink 2-3 times a day.

OTHER NATURAL TREATMENTS

Enema–Mix 1 teaspoon of baking soda or the juice of 1/2 of a **fresh** lemon with seeds strained, into a bag of warm distilled or spring water. Use this solution in an enema.

COMMERCIALLY PREPARED HERBAL REMEDIES

Herbs: HAS Original Formula (for allergies, sinus, asthma and respiratory problems. Use this if you are sensitive to Pseudoephedrine.); Breath-Aid (Use only if not sensitive to Pseudoephedrine.); IF Formula (immune system); Echinacea Combination; Fenu-Thyme (Thins out and breaks up mucus.); GL Formula (Cleanses the glands.); Liveron (Cleanses the liver.); Winter Formula (For cold and flu); Herbal Influence Formula (a cold weather formula); Naturalax 2 or 3, or, Aloelax; or, Sinustop (Nature's Way).

Homeopathic: Sinus; Fever; Sore Throat; Earache; Laxative; Detoxification; Allergy; or, Cold (Natra-Bio); or, Allergy; Cold & Flu; Earache; Headache; or, Sinusitis (Medicine from Nature).

SPLINTERS

Splinters are any foreign objects that are embedded in the skin including thorns, stingers, and fragments of metal, glass, or wood.

> **WARNING:** Do not attempt to remove splinters from the eyes, or any other place that may be too dangerous or too hard to remove or may require stitches. Get immediate medical help from a doctor or hospital.

ACTION

For a simple splinter try to carefully remove the object with a disinfected needle and flat nose tweezers. Whether you can remove the object or not, wash the splintered area with a natural soap and water, apply a natural disinfectant and apply aid.

KITCHEN REMEDIES

Aloe Vera–Slice open a piece of the plant and apply the gel to the splintered area as needed to soothe the skin and fight any toxins. Or, slit open a leaf and cover the splinter, then put a bandage over it to hold it in place for about a week. Reapply daily. You may also make a juice and foment the splintered area. Covering the blades of a blender with water, turn on to a high speed, then add enough plant leaves to make a 3-6 ounces of thick juice. Apply warm liquid with a cloth or directly to the affected area. Keep moist by adding the liquid to the cloth or redampen cloth by immersion and reapply. Keep the extra in a tightly covered jar to use as needed.

Apple Cider Vinegar–Works as a good anti-infection agent. Moisten a little piece of cotton and bandage the cotton to the area overnight or for about a week. Remoisten cotton daily.

Cayenne–Speeds healing and fights any potential infections. Moisten enough powder to make a paste with water or vegetable oil, apply it to the splintered area, and cover it with a bandage. Repeat 1-2 times daily for about a week.

Meat Tenderizer–If you cannot remove a small splinter, moisten some tenderizer with a little vegetable oil and apply it to the splinter. Loosely cover the splinter with a bandage to keep it clean. Reapply daily for about a week. The bromelain from the pineapple in the meat tenderizer will help loosen the tissue without harm so the embedded object can work its way out easier.

Sage–This is a natural disinfectant and healer. Make solution of sage tea, then add 1/4 teaspoon of ginger and 1/4 teaspoon of cayenne to use as a fomentation. Keep moist by adding the liquid to the cloth or redampen cloth by immersion and reapply for about a week.

Wheat Germ Oil–Apply a little of the oil to the area, covering with a bandage to soothe the sore skin and fight infections. Reapply for about a week.

SINGLE HERBAL REMEDIES

Wood Betony–For drawing out deeply embedded splinters this is the best. Use as a fomentation and as tea to heal.

Southern Wood–Great for drawing out the splinters as a fomentation. First make a tea by putting 10-20 drops of the liquid or open 1-2 capsules in a cup of hot water. Apply the warm tea with a cloth or pour directly onto the affected area. Soak the splintered area about 15 minutes 2 times a day. Keep the cloth or skin moist by adding the tea to the cloth or redampen cloth by immersion and reapply.

Agrimony–This has a strong astringent action for drawing out splinters. As a bonus it heals wounds. Apply the warm liquid with a cloth or directly pour over the affected area. Keep moist by adding the liquid to the cloth or redampen cloth by immersion and reapply. Repeat the fomentation 1-2 times a day. If the embedded object is in the finger or toes, put the warm liquid in a pan and soak for 10-15 minutes 2-3 times a day.

Hawthorn–The crushed or steeped leaves are the best, if you can get them. However, you can also open 2 capsules and mix the contents with a little water or vegetable oil to make a thick paste and apply several times daily. This pulls out embedded thorns or splinters. As an even quicker remedy use the syrup form. Take about 1-2 teaspoons of the syrup 3 times daily and gently rub a little over the splinter 2-3 times daily. If you need to cover the splinter with a bandage, then just peal the bandage back to reapply herbal remedy and recover. If the bandage is dirty, then replace it.

COMMERCIALLY PREPARED HERBAL REMEDIES

Herbs: Cal-Silica Formula (natural calcium); Echinacea Combination Extract (A great infection fighter and antibiotic to be used by applying it to the splintered area and take.); BF&C (Rebuilds bone, flesh and cartilage.); Black ointment (Helps to remove a splinter or embedded object.) (Nature's Way); liquid trace mineral (Great for healing and knitting up wounds with out scarring. Take 1/2 ounce in 4-6 ounces of vegetable or fruit juice 2-3 times daily and apply as needed.); or, Rescue Remedy (shock and trauma) (Bach).

Homeopathic: Injuries; Fever; Insect Bites; or, Pain (Natra Bio).

SPRAINS

Sprains involve damaged ligaments without a dislocation or fracture occurring. They generally swell and are painful. These occur when a joint is forced to move past its usual range of motion.

ACTION

Use ice or a cold water compress for about 5 minutes at a time. Then rest for an interval of 15 minutes before reapplying ice or cold water for another 5 minutes. You can also alternate warm water for 20-30 minutes, with cold water for 1 minute each hour or as needed. Also elevate the injured part and rest it. In addition, use the suggested remedies.

KITCHEN REMEDIES

Sage–You can use this kitchen herb as a tea, fomentation, or poultice to reduce the swelling and relax the body. In a cup of hot water steep 1/2-1 teaspoon of sage with 1/4 teaspoon of cinnamon and 1-2 pinches of cayenne pepper. Take 1 cup 3 times a day. Use the tea for a fomentation by applying the warm tea with a cloth or pour the tea directly to sprained muscle. Keep moist by adding the tea to the cloth or redampen cloth by immersion and reapply. As a poultice, mix the amounts given for the tea in warm olive or vegetable oil and apply to the sprain. Foment or poultice the sprain 2-3 times a week.

Apple Cider Vinegar–Works as an antispasmodic. Take 1 teaspoon of apple cider vinegar in 4-6 ounces of water. You may also wet a cotton ball or cloth to hold the vinegar on the sprained muscle for several minutes, or tape on the cloth or cotton ball. Reapply several times a day.

Olive, Castor, or Wheat Germ Oil–Mix these oils together or use them separately by rubbing them over the sprained muscle. The castor oil is for the pain and swelling while the olive and wheat germ rebuilds the tissue.

Easy Preparation of Cabbage, Carrot, or Garlic Poultice: Chop, grate, or slice the recommended vegetable or herb, then mix with vegetable or olive oil and apply to area securing the poultice with a cloth or gauze. These remedies draw out the pain and reduce the swelling. Change poultice several times daily, throwing out the used one. You can also mix the extra chopped, grated, or sliced herbs or vegetables in with other foods, soups, or juices for internal help several times daily.

SINGLE HERBAL REMEDIES

With any of the following herbal remedies you may foment the sprain as well as take the herbs internally. For fomentation apply the warm oil or liquid herb on a cloth or directly onto the sprain. Keep the cloth moist by adding a little more oil or liquid to the cloth or redampen cloth by immersion and reapply. If the sprain is easily accessible, like the wrist or foot, soak the appendage in a pan of warm herbal tea.

Ruta–Takes the swelling out. Apply as a fomentation to the sprain. The homeopathic remedy Ruta 12X is great for internal repairs.

WARNING: Do **not** take internally if pregnant.

Garlic Oil–Use ice on the area first, then a spread a light coat of olive oil before applying the garlic oil. This protects the skin from the garlic. Reduces the swelling and prevents any secondary infections from coming into the body if there is a wound as well.

Catnip–Take as a tea and apply as a fomentation. Works on the swelling and pain.

Burdock–Great for injuries especially swelling. Take as a tea and foment.

Elder Flower–Use as both a tea and fomentation.

Wintergreen Oil–This is a very strong antiseptic, relaxer, and healer. You can mix equal parts of wintergreen, any of the other herbs, and olive oil to apply as a liniment. For a children's liniment dilute with 2 parts olive oil. For internal use: Adults, take small doses at time like 5-10 drops, more effective and has less of a nauseous side effects in juice or tea; Children: 1 teaspoon diluted with a little olive or sweet almond oil 2-3 times daily.

COMMERCIALLY PREPARED HERBAL REMEDIES

Herbs: BF&C capsules or ointment (Rebuilds bones, flesh and cartilage.); Cal-Silica Formula (natural calcium for healing the nerves.); Kalmin (An anti-spasmodic that calms and heals the injury.); Ex-Stress Formula (Supports the nerves) (Nature's Way); Vegetable Calcium (Schiff); Calcium Citrate (Twin Lab); Liquid Trace Mineral

(Great for soaking and healing sprains. Soak injury with 1 tablespoon of the mineral in water. Also, take from 1 teaspoon up to 1
tablespoon in juice 1-2 times daily); or, Rescue Remedy (for shock
and trauma) (Bach).

Homeopathic: Injuries; or, Pain (Natra-Bio). See a homeopath for
Ruta 3-6X potency (Garden rue is great for healing bad sprains,
weak muscles, lameness, flexor tendons and muscles and Carpel
Tunnel Syndrome.).

STREP THROAT

Strep throat is a sore throat caused by the bacterial group A strep-
tococci. Usual symptoms, aside from a sudden sore throat, are
headache, fever, nausea, and malaise. The glands on the neck are
swollen and if you look inside the person's mouth with a flashlight
you'll notice that the throat is very red and may have whitish blotch-
es.

There is a lot of fear around strep throat. This is mainly because
of the diseases that may develop if this condition isn't treated or
doesn't resolve on its own. In truth, about a quarter of the popula-
tion are carriers of strep without any symptoms. Very often people
get treated for strep even when there is no clear evidence that the
sore throat actually is strep. Only 10 percent of sore throats show
positive strep cultures.

There is some debate as to whether antibiotics are necessary or
desired to treat strep throat. For safety sake, however, if you don't
respond to the remedies I suggest in one week, or if you have a history of glomerulonephritis (a kidney disease) or rheumatic fever,
then see your doctor.

ACTION

The most important action is to rest the throat and stay warm. Drink
plenty of water and juices. Keep the bowels open. Any sore throat
tells you the colon is sluggish. Gargling with warm salt water and/or
suggested herbs is helpful.

KITCHEN REMEDIES

Apple Cider Vinegar–Acts as a disinfectant. Drink 1/4 teaspoon of apple cider vinegar in a cup of warm water several times a day. You may also gargle with the vinegar as needed.

Buttermilk or Yogurt–Both of these are natural antiseptics. Take 1 teaspoon to 1 tablespoon each hour, allowing it to trickle down throat. Do not drink any liquids for at least 30 minutes so that the butter milk or yogurt's effect is not washed away. Good for early stages of a sore throat and is great for babies and young children.

Garlic or Onion–Either works as an antiseptic. Chop, dice, or grate either or combine both together for a tea or gargle taking 2-3 times a day. In a cup of hot water mix 1/2-1 teaspoon of the vegetable with 1/4 teaspoon of cinnamon and 1-2 pinches of cayenne.

Sage–This is a good cleanser and infection fighter. Make a tea to take as well as using it for a gargle and fomentation. Apply warm liquid herb with a cloth or directly to the neck.

SINGLE HERBAL REMEDIES

Garlic Oil–This is a great cleanser and antiseptic that relieves toxins. Make a tea by putting 5-8 drops of the oil in a cup of hot or room temperature water. Drink 2-3 times a day.

Pau d'Arco–Works as both an antiseptic and antibiotic. Take about 10-20 drops in about 4-6 ounces of vegetable or fruit juice several times daily.

Echinacea–Stimulates the immune system, especially the white blood cells, and lymph glands. Works great for strep throat. Make a tea. Works well when combined with goldenseal.

WARNING: Don't take goldenseal when you're pregnant. Do not take as a single herb if you have hypoglycemia.

Figwort–Works as a good remedy for strep throat. Drink the tea and use it as a fomentation.

OTHER NATURAL TREATMENTS

Vitamin C–This vitamin was used during the 1930s to treat strep throat, before the advent of antibiotics. Take one gram of vitamin C three times a day.

COMMERCIALLY PREPARED REMEDIES

Herbs: Kalmin (anti-spasmodic); Ex-Stress (Calms the nervous system.); GL Formula (Cleanses glands and lymph nodes.); IF Formula (Supports the immune system.); Fenu-Thyme Formula (Cleans out mucus and infections,); Red Clover Combination (Nature's Way); liquid trace mineral (A great healer than can be mixed 2-3 ounces with 2-3 ounces of warm water for a gargle. Take half an ounce in vegetable or diluted fruit juice several times daily as needed. Or moisten cloth with mineral and wrap throat pinning a warm cloth around the neck. Re-moisten several times throughout the day as needed.)

Homeopathic: Fever; Laxative; Detoxification; Sore Throat; Headache and Pain; (Natra-Bio).

STROKES

A stroke could also be called a brain attack. Like a heart attack, it occurs when the blood supply to the brain is greatly diminished due to a clot or a ruptured blood vessel. Strokes usually occur in the elderly whose arteries have hardened or high blood pressure is a problem.

The signs of a stroke, also known as apoplexy or a cerebrovascular accident, can include unconsciousness, paralysis or weakness on one side of the body, trouble breathing and swallowing, slurred or the inability to speak, confusion, loss of bladder and bowel control, and unequal pupil size.

WARNING: This is a serious problem and you should get the individual to the hospital as soon as possible.

ACTION

Use any of the recommended remedies while seeking emergency help. Make sure the person is breathing. Use CPR if necessary (See "Heart Attack"). Turn the person on his side so any secretions will drain out and not choke him. Do not give anything by mouth if he's unconscious, or stop if he starts vomiting.

STY

A sty is an infection of various glands surrounding the eye. It begins with tenderness, redness, and pain along the edge of the eyelid. With time, the infection causes tearing and sensitivity to light. Swelling occurs and yellow spots of pus appear. When these spots pop and drain, the pain decreases.

ACTION

Carefully and gently clean the area by first washing the area of the sty with a natural soap and water. Then disinfect the sty with a natural disinfectant.

In addition, drink plenty of good water, take walks, and do some eye movement exercises and apply aid. If the problem with the sty continues check with a doctor.

KITCHEN REMEDIES

Aloe Vera Plant–Clip a little piece off the end of a leaf. Squeeze a small drop into the corner of the eye near the nose while sitting or lying. Then, turn the head so the aloe gel slides into the eye and blink the eye a few times. Do the other eye if needed. The aloe will soothe the eye and bathe the sty to clear it. Repeat a few times daily, especially at bedtime and leave in overnight. The plant piece will automatically re-seal itself daily, so just puncture the sealed tip with a knife or pin to get more aloe drops.

Onions–Another help is to chop onions to bring out the tears so that the eyes can be moistened and drained. You can also place a nice size slice of onion over the closed eye with the sty to draw out the infection for a few minutes. Be sure to gently wash the affected eye where the onion laid afterwards.

Sage–Pour hot water over 1/2 teaspoon of sage in cup of water, steep for one minute with saucer on top. Allow solution to cool to room temperature. Moisten a cotton ball or a soft cloth with solution and place on the sty for about 10 minutes a few times a day. You can also soak the eye with 1/2 cup of the tea solution in an eye cup for about 5 minutes. Save the extra tea solution in a cool place and repeat as needed.

Olive Oil–With an eye dropper or a finger, place 1 drop of oil in the corner of the eye next to the nose. Close the infected eye for about 5 minutes, then wipe the oil off with a dry cloth, tissue or cotton ball.

SINGLE HERBAL REMEDIES

Burdock Root–One of the best blood purifiers. Take 1 teaspoon or 2 capsules 3-4 times daily.

Red Raspberry or Marshmallow–Red raspberry has drawing powers while marshmallow is very soothing especially for inflamed conditions like a sty. Make a tea by putting 10-20 drops of each or combine in equal parts or 1 capsule of each or 2 capsules of the singular herb in a cup of hot or room temperature water, or in juice. Drink 2-3 times a day.

Fennel or Myrrh–Myrrh is a powerful antimicrobial and fennel assists in healing sties. Make a tea by putting 10-20 drops of each or combine in equal parts or 1 capsule of each or 2 capsules of the singular herb in a cup of hot or room temperature water, or in juice. Drink 2-3 times a day.

Echinacea–Supports the immune system and purifies the blood. Make a tea and drink.

Sarsaparilla or Mullein–Sarsaparilla balances the body while mullein soothes inflammation. Foment eye for 1 hour 3-4 times daily or overnight and drink some tea. Make a tea by putting 10-20 drops of each or combine in equal parts or 1 capsule of each or 2 capsules of the singular herb in a cup of hot or room temperature water, or in juice. Drink 2-3 times a day.

OTHER NATURAL TREATMENTS

Hot/Cold Packs–Use these packs to bring a sty to a head and to draw pus out. Alternate hot/cold packs over eye. One minute for cold and 3 minutes for hot. Can use small hot/cold thermal bags from drug store. One filled with cold water and or ice and the other with warm water. If you do not have thermal bags, use hot and cold water in a wash cloth squeezed out and placed over the eye for a few minutes. Be careful not to burn yourself with the hot pack.

COMMERCIALLY PREPARED REMEDIES

Herbs: Eyebright (Use this herb for an eye wash.); Eyebright Combination; Liveron (A good liver cleaner.); Cal-Silica (Nature's Way); or liquid trace minerals.

Homeopathic: Eye Irritation; Pain; Injuries; or Cold Sores/Fever Blisters (Natra-Bio).

SUNBURN

Sunburn generally happens to people who have not been out in the sun for a while, then decide they need a tan, trying to do it quickly over a weekend. Damage to the skin due to heat and the sun's rays can cause a reddening of the skin with mild swelling and pain in mild sunburn cases, similar to first-degree burns.

A second-degree burn from a very deep sunburn can be more severe and more painful and may display light to heavy blisters with deep redness. This can cause considerable swelling over a period of several days with a wet appearance on the surface of the skin because of the loss of plasma through the damaged layers of the skin.

Try to use natural sun screen blockers, like aloe vera gel or zinc oxide, across the nose over to the ears and on the shoulders. Reapply several times during the outing, especially if you go into any water. It's best to build up the skin's exposure to the sun slowly. Begin with a daily exposure of 10-20 minutes a day.

> **WARNING:** If the burns are severe looking and extremely painful, as in a second degree burn resulting from long exposure to the sun, see your physician.

ACTION

First-aid is intended to relieve the pain of first or second-degree burns because usually these do not require medical treatment. Just apply cold water or submerge the burn area in cold water (**not** ice water) until the pain stops. Then apply cloth wrung out in ice water and blot the skin dry, gently. Do not break any blisters. You can apply a natural antiseptic cream, ointment, or a gel like aloe vera gel from a prepared bottle or the plant. Cover the area with the selected cream, ointment or other suggested remedies as gently as possible using clean hands, a piece of cotton, or any other applicator.

KITCHEN REMEDY

Aloe Vera–Cut a piece of the plant and apply directly to the sunburn several times daily. You can use a fresh slice 1-2 times per day or overnight as needed.

Sage–Make a tea to gently apply on the sunburn by either using soft cotton or putting the tea in a spray bottle and spraying. You may also drink 1-3 cups daily to help with dehydration. In a cup of water mix 1 teaspoon of sage, 1/4 teaspoon of cinnamon and 1-2 pinches of cayenne.

Apple Cider Vinegar–This takes the sting out from a sunburn. Just carefully spray or wipe the sunburn with some vinegar as needed.

Witch Hazel–Take 1 teaspoon 3 times daily in juice and apply to the sunburn with a cotton or put some in a spray bottle and spray on. Apply every 1-2 hours or as needed. Witch Hazel tones, moistens and disinfects the skin.

Honey and/or Olive, or Wheat Germ Oil–Take 1/2 teaspoon 2-3 times a day with water or juice to help keep the skin moist. Lightly spread any of these remedies over the burned area. You may use the honey or either oil separately or in combination.

Potato or Onions–Use either one or in combination as a poultice.

SINGLE HERBAL REMEDIES

Bayberry–This is especially good for a slow healing sunburn. Make a tea. Drink 2-3 times a day to heal quicker. Apply as a fomentation the warm liquid with a cloth or directly to the sunburn by using a spray bottle. Keep moist by adding the liquid to the cloth or redampen cloth by immersion and reapply several times daily.

Calendula–Good for all types of sunburns and heals the skin's damaged nerve endings. You may add this herb to any of the other herbs listed for speedier nerve healing. Make a tea.

Drink the tea 2-3 times a day as well as using as a fomentation. Apply the warm tea with a piece of cotton or put it in spray bottle and spray directly onto the sunburn. Keep moist by adding the tea to the cloth or redampen cloth by immersion and reapply, or, spray the area as needed.

OTHER NATURAL TREATMENTS

Vitamin E (200-400 IU)–Take 1 capsule daily and apply to the sunburn as it will speed healing. Puncture a perle, then squeeze the content out and spread it over the sunburn.

WARNING: Avoid vitamin E supplementation if you are taking blood thinning medication or if you have liver disease.

COMMERCIALLY PREPARED HERBAL REMEDIES

Herbs: For 1st and 2nd degree burns, apply right away and often BF&C or Comfrey ointments for external use; or, Silent Night (Aids rest and sleep.) (Nature's Way); or, Rescue Remedy (for shock and trauma) (Bach). Particularly great is Liquid Trace Mineral as it speeds up healing particularly if it is sprayed on right away for 10-20 minutes every 1-2 hours. Also add about 1/2 ounce of mineral in fruit (apple juice) 3-5 times daily until better and gradually reduce amount.

Homeopathic: Detoxification; Injuries; Neuralgic Pains; Pain; Fever; or, Exhaustion (Natra-Bio); Fatigue; Insomnia; or, Headache (Medicine from Nature); Calms (Hylands).

For second degree sunburns it is best to use Cantharis 30-200X. Take 2 tablets and spray area every 30 minutes every 1-2 hours. To make the spray, dissolve 6-8 tablets in 1 quart of spring water in a spritz bottle, shake to dissolve and shake the mix before each spraying of the area. If using liquid add about 20-30 drops of 30-200X potency in 1 quart of spring water in a spray bottle, applying to the burns every 30 minutes to every 1-2 hours. Slightly warm up either spray formula before applying. I used this remedy and technique on a 3rd degree explosion burn and healed the infected area in about 5-7 days with no scarring.

You can also follow up with hypericum and calendula ointment and tablets for painful burns as it prevents scaring and reduces nerve pain. Make a spray according to directions for a Cantharis spray. This is especially good for preventing muscle and nerve damage (Boericke & Tafel). Also see a homeopath if further help is required.

SWOLLEN GLANDS

Glandular swelling occurs in the lymph nodes due to infection and congestion. The areas of the body most effected are the breast, thyroid, neck, testes, groin, and under the jaw and arms.

This condition is when there is enlargement, congestion, tenderness, or the soreness of the lymph nodules anywhere in the body.

However, the areas most affected are in the neck, breast, under the arms, groin, and testes. Lymphatic swelling is usually due to bacteria or other infections in the body, and, a residue often causes lymph filtering nodes to become clogged and sluggish in it's filtering job.

The lympathic system is the first line of defense of the body against infections, that may need more water and cleansing herbs to clear out the mucus, virus, and bacteria.

> **WARNING:** Chronically swollen glands could be the result of something serious like AIDS and some types of cancer. If this is the case, visit with your doctor.

ACTION

Try to determine cause of swelling like a cold, flu, or infection. Take and apply the suggested remedies.

Get more rest, drink plenty of water, eat better food, or try a liquid fast for few days. Keep bowels open, and some do a light exercise, like walking or bouncing on a rebounder and apply remedy. Check if a flu or cold is involved in the congestion of the bowels.

KITCHEN REMEDIES

Spiced Sage Tea–Make sage tea to fight the toxins by adding 1/4 teaspoon of cinnamon with a pinch of ginger. Drink every 1-2 hours. Also use sage with a pinch of cayenne powder and garlic.

Apple Cider Vinegar–Dilute 1 tablespoon in 32 ounces of water or juice and drink 4-6 ounces throughout the day to help clean the infections from the system and glands, healing and cleansing tonic. Also, you can rub some onto the swollen area.

Castor or Olive Oil–Either one of these oils, or both combined break down the congestion and infection, relieves pain. Gently rub the swollen area with warm oil several times daily and overnight. Wrap the area well with a cloth or towel, and, if you wish, you can lay a heating pad on the swollen area for about 10-20 minutes at a time. Do 2 to 3 times per day. Be sure to stay covered and warm afterwards. For extra help add some garlic to the oils.

Parsley–Chop and steep a good handful of parsley in a pint of hot water for 5-10 minutes. Strain and drink, hot or cold, 4-6 ounces throughout the day until the pint is finished. Repeat as needed. This is a good natural diuretic that cleans the liver, gall bladder, adrenals, and any other swollen and enlarged glands.

> **WARNING:** Very large doses of parsley leaf may cause nerve damage, bleeding in the gut, liver damage, and abortion.

Garlic and Onion–Separately chop, grate, or juice both vegetables. Then combine 1/4 teaspoon of each in a cup of warm tea or juice. Drink every 1-2 hours. Both of these vegetables are antibiotics and antiseptics. You may also make a poultice and apply heat with a heating pad covered with a towel to protect the skin.

Horseradish–Take 1/2 teaspoon of prepared horseradish eventually working up to 1 teaspoon 2-3 times daily. Hold it in mouth or eat a little in food. If fresh root is available, grate it very finely and soak it in apple juice or olive oil for a few days with fresh diced garlic. Put this mixture in a tight sealed jar and store in refrigerator. When needed either take directly into the mouth or mix it with some food or juice, gradually increasing the amount until you are use to it. Works great as an antiseptic, decongestant, and cleansing tonic.

SINGLE HERBAL REMEDIES

Thyme–This is a powerful antiseptic and healing tonic. In addition, you can mix fenugreek with the thyme in the same proportions or buy the already prepared combination. Use as a fomentation as well as a tea.

Mullein–As a hot tea it is a great remedy for swollen lymph nodes due to its anti-inflammatory actions.

Echinacea–Purifies the blood of the infection. Echinacea may be combined with any of the listed remedies to speed healing by adding 10-15 drops or taking 1-2 capsules. Make a tea.

Marshmallow–Releases mucus and phlegm, and acts as a powerful anti-inflammatory. This can be used effectively as a fomentation and tea.

Oak Bark–An excellent herb for healing swollen glands. For sore throats use this as a gargle, tea, and fomentation.

Bayberry–This raises the vitality and resistance of the body by working as a circulatory stimulant. Make a tea.

Wheat Germ Oil–Gently rub the wheat germ oil onto the sore area to clean out the toxins and speed healing. Then cover with a cloth and apply heat.

Witch Hazel–Spread over the swollen glands.

Gland Cleansing Tea–This combination fights infections and cleans the lymph system. Mix in a cup of hot water, 1/4-1/2 teaspoon of goldenseal, echinacea, and mullein. Drink the tea 2-3 times a day as needed.

Goldenseal–Make a tea with this immune system stimulant.

OTHER NATURAL TREATMENTS

Compresses–Alternate hot and cold compresses to the swelling gland. Leave the hot compress on for about 1-2 minutes at a time, and the cold for about 30 seconds. To do a compress you may use either hot towels or a heating pad.

Soak Baths–A great relaxing tonic for the whole body. The heat encourages the release of toxins through the skin. While filling the tub with hot water suited to your body add single or combination of herbs desired. Tinctured or liquid teas are very good here. You can also use steeped bulk tea here or place some bulk herbs in a clean sock tied at the end. Use 1-2 cups of epsom salts or 1 cup of aloe vera, apple cider vinegar, or baking soda.

Vitamin E (400 IU) or A (10,000 IU)–Take E and A daily. Also, puncture capsules and apply to the swollen area. As antioxidants, either vitamin is a good cleanser for congested lymph nodes.

WARNING: Avoid vitamin E supplementation if you are talking blood thinning medication or if you have liver disease.

COMMERCIALLY PREPARED HERBAL REMEDIES

Herbs: GL Formula (for lungs and glands); IF Formula (Supports the immune system.); Myrrh-Golden Seal Plus (for various infections); Echinacea Combination (Improves overall immunity.); Fenu-Thyme Formula (Cleans out mucus and lymph glands.) (Nature's Way); or, liquid trace mineral (Take 1/2 ounce in 4-6 ounces of vegetable or fruit juice several times daily. Also soak area several times daily if infected.).

Homeopathic: Flu; Cold; Earache; Sore Throat; Sinus; Laxative; Detoxification; or, Pain (Natra-Bio.); or, Cold & Flu; Earache; or, Fatigue (Medicine from Nature).

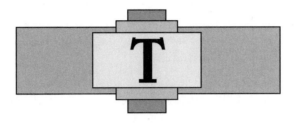

TEETHING

You know a baby is teething when she begins gnawing or chewing on her hands or anything else, drools a lot, or becomes irritable—crying, whining, cranky, or restless. Other symptoms may include a fever, diarrhea, congestion, spitting up, runny nose, stuffiness, and reddish gums.

> **WARNING:** Do not give children alcohol based tinctures. Do not give children less than one year old honey either straight or as a sweetener in any herbal preparations.

ACTION

For prevention give any of the suggested remedies to your child before teething begins as well as during the crisis. If the mother is breast feeding, she can take the remedies to help protect her system and provide more free calcium and phosphorus through her milk to the baby. Enemas help remove toxins from the body. Chinese medicine draws a line between the bowels and lungs, thus enemas also help drain excess mucus from the lungs. This helps prevent infections. If you need further help contact your local homeopath.

KITCHEN REMEDIES

Sage–Calms the baby's nerves and assists the budding teeth to come through the gums. Mix 1/4 teaspoon of sage powder in a cup of hot water with 1/4 teaspoon of catnip, adding a little sweetener like maple syrup for taste. Cool this solution before giving it to your child in a baby bottle 2-3 times a day or as needed. You may also use warm juice instead of water. If you are a nursing mother, do not take sage as this herb dries up breast milk.

Cayenne–Cayenne is high in calcium and vitamin C, and is an antiseptic. Vitamin C is effective for injured tissues. Mix 1-2 pinches with a little glycerine and rub onto the gums. In addition, you may give 1/16 teaspoon in a bottle of water, juice, or milk 3-4 times daily.

Wheat Germ Oil–Mix with a little glycerine and rub onto the gums. Give a little of the wheat germ oil straight or put a 1/4 teaspoon in a bottle 3-4 times daily.

SINGLE HERBAL REMEDIES

Catnip, Fennel, or Clove Oil–Add 2-5 drops of either a single herb or mix equal parts of all three in a bottle, adding a little maple syrup for taste. Also rub the herbal mixture on the baby's gums as needed. These herbs calm the baby's nerves and keep her gums from becoming inflamed while her teeth are coming through.

Chamomile–Settles the baby's nerves. This tea is also great for the mother who is at her wit's end taking care of a crying baby. Give 5-10 drops 1-3 times daily either straight or in bottle of water or juice. And rub onto gums.

Red Raspberry–Provides some calcium and vitamin C. It's astringent property eases gum pain. Give 5-10 drops of oil, empty 1 capsule, or 1/2 teaspoon of the liquid into a bottle of water or juice. Drink 1-3 times daily. Rub on gums. Great for diarrhea and fever that may accompany teething.

COMMERCIALLY PREPARED HERBAL REMEDIES

Herbs: Cal-Silica (natural calcium); BF&C capsules (Rebuilds bone, flesh and cartilage.); Kalmin (anti-spasmodic); any natural liquid calcium; or, phosphate with D (if possible.).

Homeopathic: Teething; Teeth & Gums; Indigestion; Neuralgic Pains; or, Detoxification (Natra Bio); Teething; Colic; Calms; or, Diarrhea (Hyland); Teething; Colic; Earache; Indigestion & Gas; Insomnia; Sinusitis (Medicine from Nature); Calcium Carbonate (Take 2 tablets, 3-6X potency, every 2-4 hours as needed.); or, lime water (Take as directed. Helps calcium absorption to enable the new teeth to come through quicker and easier.).

TEETH GRINDING (BRUXISM)

Bruxism is the unconscious grinding or clenching of teeth often during sleep. This can occur as a result of too much stress. Sometimes poor calcium absorption or intake can contribute to this problem as this mineral feeds the nerves and muscles. This condition also increases as you get older. Chronic bruxism can eventually erode the tops of teeth and even loosen them. Other times the person may notice that his jaw is sore, especially in the morning. While many people are unaware of this habit, those around them do notice it.

ACTION

Improve your diet by eating more calcium enriched foods such as yogurt and other dairy products, and dark leafy green vegetables like spinach and kale, and drink more water. Use the suggested remedies. If stress is a factor, use some relaxation techniques. See "Insomnia."

KITCHEN REMEDIES

Sage–Sage helps relieve spasming or tense muscles in the jaw. Make a tea with the powder or leaves adding 1/4 teaspoon of catnip. Be sure to drink a cup of tea 2 hours before bedtime.

Catnip, Chamomile, Peppermint, or Spearmint–These sedative herbs calm and relax the body. Some also soothe tense jaw muscles. You can even find these herbs as teas in the grocery or health food store already prepared. However, if you have or only can find the loose leaf herbs make a tea.

Apple Cider Vinegar–Calms the body. Take 1/2 teaspoon of apple cider vinegar in a cup of hot water, then drink it and go to bed.

Milk–For this remedy it is best to use goat, whey, or skimmed milk. Drink a glass of warm milk before bed as a sedative. The calcium in milk is also beneficial for the teeth, muscles, and nerves.

SINGLE HERBAL REMEDIES

Horsetail Grass–Make a tea and drink 2-3 times a day.

Oat Straw–Oats are useful in cases of nervous exhaustion and general debility. It's also very nutritious when eaten as oatbran or oatmeal. Make a tea and drink 2-3 times a day.

COMMERCIALLY PREPARED HERBAL REMEDIES

Herbs: Cal-Silica Formula (natural calcium); BF&C capsules (Rebuilds bone, flesh and cartilage,); Kalmin (anti-spasmodic); Ex-Stress Extract (great for calming and feeding nervous system); Bone All (Schiff); Calcium Citrate (Twin Lab); or, Rescue Remedy (for shock and trauma) (Bach).

Homeopathic: Calcium Carbonate, 6-12X potency (Aids calcium absorption.); Teeth and Gums; Neuralgic Pains; Earache; or, Pain (Natra Bio); Teething; Calms. For further help see a homeopath.

TOENAIL, INGROWN

An ingrown toenail is a nail that grows downward into the skin causing pain and infection that could lead to a more serious infection if not taken care of properly. My theory is this problem is usually due to poor calcium and silicon intake or absorption, or possibly poor circulation.

ACTION

Wash the ingrown toenail with a natural soap and water. Then use a natural disinfectant. After cleaning the toenail you can lift the inward growing toenail if it is not too deep or infected. Take a small peace of cotton and carefully slide it under the edge of the nail with a fingernail file, or tweezers. This may be painful if the nail is deep into the skin so you may have to raise the nail slowly a little at a time each day. This method prevents the nail from growing further into the skin and causing other infections. You may leave the cotton under the nail to gently allow the nail to grow upwards naturally without pain. And, this makes it easier to disinfect the deeper tissue with natural disinfects or hydrogen peroxide and applying a healing remedy. I have corrected several nail problems in this natural way.

Additional calcium may help the nail to grow correctly. Check the nail for discoloration as you may need an antifungal remedy as well (see the "Fungus" section.) Also, never cut the nail rounded, but straight across and not close into the skin. If toenail looks or becomes to involved or infected see a doctor before problem becomes worse.

KITCHEN REMEDIES

Aloe Vera Plant–To fight infection, to soothe the painful toe, and speed healing, cut small piece from the leaf of a plant, slice it open, and apply to the toenail. Use a bandage to secure it to the toe. You may sprinkle a little garlic or cayenne onto the gel to fight an infection. You can also purchase aloe vera liquid or gel from a health food store to use on the toenail or to drink. Take 1-2 teaspoons 1-2 times daily in juice for additional antibiotic effect.

Apple Cider Vinegar–Dab the vinegar with a piece of cotton directly onto the toenail to disinfect it and soothe the pain. If it is too strong, dilute and cover the toe with a bandage.

Castor or Olive Oil–First, to break up the infection rub the castor oil in and around the toenail 2-3 times daily for a few days, then apply olive oil to rebuild the tissue around the toe for a few days.

Sage–Sage can be used as a tea and poultice for an ingrown toenail to fight infection and to soothe nerves and skin. Place 1/2 teaspoon of sage in a cup of hot water and drink 2 times a day. Apply to the toenail as poultice by mixing some olive oil with enough of the herb to cover the nail. Cover with a bandage and leave it alone. Gently replace the poultice about once a week.

Wheat Germ Oil–Take 1 teaspoon of this antiseptic 1-2 times daily and apply the oil to the toenail.

SINGLE HERBAL REMEDIES

Plantain–This wound healer comes in an ointment to speed the healing of the damaged toe tissues. Take 2 capsules or make a tea by opening capsules into a cup of hot or room temperature water, or in juice. Drink 2-3 times a day. In addition you may make a paste by mixing the powder of 2 capsules with a little olive oil and apply to the ingrown toenail. Cover the toe with a bandage.

OTHER NATURAL TREATMENTS

Vitamin E (200 IU) and A (5,000 IU)–Take 2 times daily and apply one or both in equal amounts to the area to aid healing and soothe the tenderness.

> **WARNING:** Do not take more than 50,000 IU of vitamin A per day. Avoid vitamin E supplementation if you are taking blood thinning medication or if you have liver disease.

COMMERCIALLY PREPARED HERBAL REMEDIES

Herbs: Cal-Silica Formula (natural calcium); BF&C capsules or ointment (Rebuilds bones, flesh, cartilage and nails.); Vegetable Calcium (Schiff's); Bone All (Schiff); Calcium Citrate (Rebuilds nerves and tissues) (Twin Lab); or, liquid trace mineral (great infection fighter and healer).

Homeopathic: Injuries; Headache & Pain; Emotional; Detoxification; or, Pain (Natra Bio); Injury & Backache; or, Headache (Medicine From Nature).

TONSILS (QUINSY)

Tonsils are the first line of our body's defense system to protect it against infections. Quinsy, also known as peritonsillar abscesses, is one type of infection that strikes tonsils. This severe inflammation of the tonsils and peritonsillar tissues usually appear red with swelling, and pus (peritonsillar abscess). Other symptoms are fever, chills, pain in swallowing, a swollen throat and tongue, a dry mouth, and there may be difficulty in breathing if the throat swells. Although strep is the usual cause of quinsy, other germs can cause it too. (See "Strep throat.") Quinsy usually strikes young adults; it's uncommon in children. Remember: Sore throat, dirty colon.

ACTION

Improve the diet by eating more fruit, roughage, and vegetables. Drink more fluids, like soups as well as water, to keep bowels and kidneys functioning optimally. Avoid sugar intake.

KITCHEN REMEDIES

Ginger–This is a good sweating and cleansing herb. Make a tea using 1/4-1/2 teaspoon of the spice. Great to combine in equal parts with sage. Take 2-3 times a day and gargle with it as needed.

Sage–A good cleanser of infections and swelling when used as a tea and gargle. Mix 1/2-1 teaspoon of sage for the tea adding 1/4 teaspoon of cayenne for speedier healing. Gargle with this tea several times a day.

SINGLE HERBAL REMEDIES

Bayberry–Use as an infection fighter and blood cleanser due to its astringent qualities. You may take as a tea, gargle, and foment the neck. Make a tea and drink 2-3 times a day. To foment apply warm liquid with a cloth or directly to the swollen glands. Keep moist by adding the liquid to the cloth or redampen cloth by immersion and reapply.

Black Walnut–This extract works as an infection fighter and antiseptic, blood cleanser and helps to reduce mucous. Take as a tea and foment around neck as needed. Make a tea.

Marshmallow–Marshmallow soothes inflamed tissues such as those affected in quinsy. Make a tea and drink 2-3 times a day.

Mullein–A great tonic for the mucous membranes and inflammation fighter. Take and foment. Make a tea and drink 2-3 times a day.

Red Raspberry–Works as an antiviral and antibacterial that is good for fighting fevers, mucus, and nausea. Make a tea or take the capsules 2-3 times a day.

COMMERCIALLY PREPARED HERBAL REMEDIES

Herbs: GL Formula (for inflamed glands and lymph nodes); IF Formula (Boosts immune system.); Kalmin (antispasmodic); Liveron (Cleanses the liver and gall bladder); Ex-Stress Extract (Calms and feeds the nervous system.); Naturalax 1, 2, or 3, or, Aloelax (Nature's Way); or, Liquid Trace Mineral (Great all purpose healing aid, for sore throat and tonsils, by moistening a cloth with the mineral and wrapping it around the neck. Do this several times daily. Also take 1/2 ounce in 4-6 ounces of vegetable or fruit juice several times daily.).

Homeopathic: Fever; Sore Throat; Ear Ache; Head Cold; Headache & Pain; Laxative; Flu; Teething; Candida Yeast; Detoxification; or,

Pain (Natra Bio); Cold & Flu; Earache; or, Sinusitis (Medicine From Nature).

TOOTHACHE

Most of us have experienced a toothache at one time or another. Localized pain that is dull or shooting, aching, or throbbing is usually due to a cavity, lost filling, or other local infection in or around that tooth. This is particularly true if you also experience sensitivity to cold, hot, or sweets in that area. Occasionally other conditions can cause toothaches such as allergies, an infection of the salivary gland, quinsy, skin infection or, in my experience, a build up of toxins in the body.

ACTION

It is best to see your dentist when you can. In the meantime, brush you teeth thoroughly, checking for any further food residue by flossing. Sometimes the pain will greatly reduce when food or, particularly, candy residue is removed. Apply one of the suggested remedies below directly to the toothache. Also pack calcium and cayenne directly to painful area.

KITCHEN REMEDIES

Cayenne–One of the fastest and best tooth pain relievers available. If you have fresh peppers use them, otherwise pack the tooth with the powder. Unless the tooth is greatly infected, cayenne pepper will not burn the mucus in the area of the sore tooth. My wife woke up at 2:00 A.M. with a bad toothache, she packed the area with cayenne and in 5 minutes was able to go back to sleep. Take a handful of pepper and mix in a enough water or vegetable oil to make a paste, then mold it around the inflamed tooth. You can also drink a tea with 1-2 pinches of cayenne mixed in a cup of warm water. This will equalize the blood throughout the head and body, relieving the head and toothache. If the tea doesn't relieve the aching, then add more cayenne to the next cup.

Apple Cider Vinegar–Warm the vinegar, then hold it in the mouth near the tooth or use a piece of cotton to foment the sore tooth. Apply warm liquid with a cloth or cotton swab to the sore tooth. Or, hold the solution on the side of the mouth where the toothache is. Keep the cloth or swab moist by adding the liquid to either or redampen by immersion and reapply.

Sage–Use as a poultice or make a tea, using a 1/2 teaspoon of sage, for drinking and holding the solution in the mouth. Adding a little cayenne is helpful.

Cloves–If possible use fresh cloves. Steep 1 tablespoon for 20 minutes in 2 cups of water. Cool and apply with a piece of cotton to hold solution to the tooth. Or, suck on several cloves. These are also good as breath fresheners.

Garlic–Make a poultice to apply to the tooth to fight the infection. And you can also take some of the garlic in a little juice or in a cup of hot water.

Chamomile, Cinnamon, or Ginger–Take any of these as an antiseptic teas and use on the sore tooth, or pack tooth area. Make a tea with 1/4-1/2 teaspoon of the herb or spices and drink. Cool the tea and apply with a piece of cotton to hold solution to the tooth. Mix the herb or spices in a enough water or vegetable oil to make a paste, then mold it around the inflamed tooth.

Thyme–This is a great antiseptic against tooth decay. Either rub the tea directly onto the tooth or pack the area. Use 1/4-1/2 of a teaspoon of thyme in the tea preparation explained above. Mix the herb in a enough water or vegetable oil to make a paste, then mold it around the inflamed tooth.

SINGLE HERBAL REMEDIES

Clove Oil or Camphor–Foment the aching tooth. Apply warm liquid with a cloth or directly to the affected area by holding the solution in the mouth. Keep moist by adding the liquid to the cloth or redampen cloth by immersion and reapply.

> **WARNING:**   Large doses are toxic to children. Don't use camphor oil on children.

Sassafras Oil–Dilute oil with a little olive oil and rub the oil directly onto the tooth or pack the area to fight the infection. Apply the warm oil mixture with a piece for cloth around the tooth. Keep moist by adding the oil to the cloth or redampen cloth by immersion and reapply. You can also drink as a tea. Use 5 to 10 drops of oil in juice or open 1-2 capsules in a cup of hot water. Drink 3-4 times a day.

Garlic Oil–This works as a natural antibiotic and anti-infection fighter. Use as a tea, rub the oil directly to the infected tooth or pack area. Make a tea by putting 5-8 drops of the oil in a cup of hot or room temperature water. Drink 2-3 times a day. To pack the tooth, apply warm tea or the undiluted oil with a piece of cloth to put on the tooth. Keep moist by adding the liquid to the cloth or redampen cloth by immersion and reapply.

Calendula–This is the natural "first-aid" herb for teeth and earaches that can occur from a tooth problem. Make a tea and drink 2-3 times a day. You may also rub the sore tooth area with some of the tea or pack the tooth by applying the warm tea to a piece of cloth to put on the tooth. Keep the cloth moist by adding the tea to the cloth.

Black Walnut–The extract kills infection and helps restore tooth enamel. Make a tea.

Peppermint Oil–Take as an antiseptic tea and rub either on the tooth or pack area. Make a tea by putting 5-10 drops of the oil in juice or open 1-2 capsules in a cup of hot or room temperature water. Drink 3-4 times a day. Apply warm liquid with a piece of cloth around the tooth. Keep moist by adding the liquid to the cloth or redampen cloth by immersion and reapply.

OTHER NATURAL TREATMENTS

Cool Pack–Use either an ice bag or put ice in a plastic baggy and apply to jaw area as needed.

Hot/Cold Soak–Put one foot in hot water and the other in cold for a 3 minute foot bath. Do this several times as needed. This pulls the blood and poisons away from the head area and reduces the pressure.

COMMERCIALLY PREPARED HERBAL REMEDIES

Herbs: Kalmin (antispasmodic); Cal-Silica Formula (natural calcium); Ex-Stress Extract (Calms the nervous system); Echinacea Combination (infection fighter); Bone Meal (Schiff's); Calcium Citrate (for tissues and nerves) (Twin Lab); Rescue Remedy (for shock and trauma) Bach); or, Liquid Trace Mineral (Great infection fighter and healer that can be either held in the mouth or packed in with moist cotton against the sore tooth several times daily. Also take 1/2 ounce of mineral in 4-6 ounces of vegetable or fruit juice several times daily. Call your dentist.)

Homeopathic: Toothache; Headache & Pain; Injuries; Neuralgic Pains; Earache; Insomnia; Teeth & Gums; or, Pain (Natra Bio); Calms (Hylands); Earache; Insomnia; Sinusitis; (Medicine From Nature).

TRAUMATIC SHOCK

There are many different types of shock. What they all have in common is a depression of the vital body functions due because of greatly reduced blood flow.

In this chapter, I'm going to focus on traumatic shock which occurs when there's a physical injury. The degree of shock depends on the seriousness of the trauma or injury such as a bad fall, accident, blow, poisoning by chemicals, alcohol or drugs, burns, surgery, heart attack, stroke, prolonged vomiting, or hemorrhaging.

The symptoms of shock can be in any combination of thirst, nausea, overall body weakness, a pale face, irregular or shallow breathing, chills, a weak and rapid pulse, and cold and clammy skin.

> **WARNING:** If the person has a serious injury, do what you can for immediate first-aid such as stopping a bleeding wound (See "Bleeding"), but be aware that shock can be very serious even leading to death. Call for emergency help immediately if the person is unconscious and cannot be revived.

ACTION

Check the injury carefully for bleeding and broken bones. If the person is seriously injured try not to move him or her, unless they are in danger as it may cause more damage.

Make the person as comfortable and warm as possible, and elevate their feet slightly, about 8 to 12 inches. Call a doctor or ambulance and apply suggested first aid. If person is unconscious or delirious, apply an antispasmodic tincture just inside the corner of the mouth in order not to choke them or rub the remedy into palm of hands, feet, or navel for absorption.

KITCHEN REMEDIES

NOTE: Do not give someone in shock anything by mouth unless professional medical help doesn't arrive for an hour. DO NOT give anything by mouth to someone AT ALL if:

> they are unconscious
> they are having convulsions
> they are vomiting
> they are likely to vomit
> they have an abdominal wound
> they are likely to have surgery
> they are likely to have an anesthetic.

Cayenne–Improves the circulation of the blood throughout the body. Make a tea. If the person is unconscious make paste with warm water or warm olive or vegetable oil and apply it to the navel, inside of the corner of the mouth, palms, or feet to help revive them.

Sage–This is a good nervine to calm system. Make a tea.

Celery–Helps to calm the body's system. Use freshly chopped celery to blend with some water to make a warm tea or juice. If fresh is not available, use the flakes.

SINGLE HERBAL REMEDIES

Shock Drink–Combine 1-2 tablespoons of apple cider vinegar, 1-2 tablespoons of honey, add 1/2 teaspoon of cayenne and about 10-15 drops of either valerian root or Kalmin extract (an antispasmodic) in a quart of warm water. Mix well. Administer 4-6 ounces of the drink for adults. Repeat as often as needed and remember to shake the mixture before taking. Keep in a cool place until needed.

Catnip–This is a great herb for calming babies and small children. Make a tea and drink 2-3 times a day.

Red Clover–Improves the blood circulation. Make a tea and drink 2-3 times a day.

Mullein–Helps to get more oxygen into the blood stream, thereby improving circulation. Mullein is a sedative. Make a tea and drink 2-3 times a day.

Peppermint or Spearmint Oil–Either one of these relaxes and calms the nervous system. You may add a little honey to the tea. Make a tea and drink 2-3 times a day.

Skullcap or Lady's Slipper–Both of these feed and relax the nerves. Make a tea and drink 2-3 times a day.

COMMERCIALLY PREPARED HERBAL REMEDIES

Herbs: Kalmin (antispasmodic extract); Ex-Stress Formula (Calms the nervous system.); Liquid Trace Minerals (A great healer that can be applied directly as needed. Take 1/2 ounce in 4-6 ounces of vegetable or fruit juices several times daily as needed.); or, Rescue Remedy (for shock and trauma) (Bach).

Homeopathic: Emotional; Injuries; Neuralgic Pains; Nervousness; or, Pain (Natra-Bio); or, Injury & Back Pain; Fatigue; Insomnia; or, Headache (Medicine from Nature).

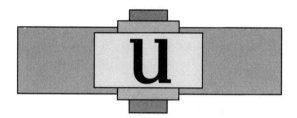

ULCERS, PEPTIC

What we usually think of when ulcers are mentioned are peptic ulcers, ones that appear in either the stomach (gastric) or small intestine (duodenal). A duodenal ulcer is more common and more painful than an often asymptomatic gastric ulcer. This irritation of the small intestine usually has a burning pain just below the breast bone, and, possibly, a bile taste in the mouth. This distress often occurs about an hour after eating and at night. Pain is intermittent and is relieved by food, antacids, or vomiting.

WARNING: If the pain is very severe or there is blood in your stools, get medical help immediately.

ACTION

Improve diet by eliminating fats and heavy meats and begin eating vegetables, fruits, soups, and broths, natural pasta, baked potatoes, cottage cheese, and buttermilk. You may take mild digestive aids. Keep the bowels open by drinking more water or liquids. And find ways to reduce excessive worry. If you smoke or take aspirin on a regular basis, eliminate these activities. Have your physician check for food allergies.

KITCHEN REMEDIES

Aloe Vera Plant–Drink aloe vera juice dilute with water or juice to soothe a peptic ulcer.

Cabbage–When using this remedy only make enough juice, 4-6 ounces, to drink immediately as it turns rancid very quickly when storing any leftovers. To make fresh cabbage juice drop the quartered pieces of cabbage to process in your juicer. Drink 2-4 times daily as needed.

Cayenne–Mix 1/4-1/2 teaspoon in a cup of hot tea, water or a little juice. Cayenne heals an internal ulcer and only burns on contact with infected mucus. If there is some burning, chew a handful or a small box of raisins. Raisins will cool the system right down. A young man came to the office having sever heartburn pains. He had a stressful job and feared being laid off. I had him drink a cup of catnip tea with a fourth teaspoon of cayenne in it twice a day for one week. Then increase the cayenne to half a teaspoon in his tea for the next month and avoid dairy products. After the first ten days his heartburn ended. He drinks the catnip tea two to three times a week as maintenance and feels great.

Baking Soda–Use this antacid if nothing else is available until a better aid is obtainable. Mix 1/4 teaspoon in 4 ounces of water, and sip slowly as needed. If while drinking the baking soda mixture, you have a burning and heat sensation, it could mean a bleeding ulcer, so contact a doctor right away.

SINGLE HERBAL REMEDIES

Burdock Root–This remedy is especially good for stomach ulcers. Take 30-50 drops or 2 capsules 3 times daily.

Chickweed–This is great for blood toxicity and inflammations especially for stomach and inflamed bowels. Take as a tea and use as a fomentation. Make a tea.

Goldenseal–Because goldenseal soothes inflamed mucous membranes, it works well for peptic ulcers. Take as a tea.

Irish Moss–For peptic ulcers, this remedy is soothing to the inflamed tissues. Irish moss also purifies and strengthens the cellular structure and vital fluids. It is high in iodine, calcium, and natural sodium, and acts as a healing agent for the stomach. Make a tea.

Calendula–A great first aid remedy that works particularly well for ulcers. Use as a soothing tea.

COMMERCIALLY PREPARED HERBAL REMEDIES

Herbs: Myrrh-Golden Seal Plus Formula (for ulcers and ulcerations); Ex-Stress Formula (Calms nervous system.); Kalmin (antispasmodic) (Nature's Way); Cabbage tablets; Ulfre (Helps ulcers and ulcerations) (Michael's); Rescue Remedy (for shock and trauma) (Bach); or, Liquid Trace Mineral (A great tissue healer that can be mixed with a 1/2 ounce of the mineral in 4-6 ounces of vegetable or fruit juice several times daily.).

Homeopathic: Nervousness; Emotional; Indigestion; Neuralgic Pains; Exhaustion; Emotional; or, Pain (Natra Bio); Indigestion & Gas.

ULCERS, SKIN

Ulcers are superficial sores with inflamed bases that discharge pus from an accumulation of dead or decaying cells. These can occur on the surface of the skin from sores or cuts on the arms or legs. Bacterial and fungal infections (See "Fungus") can also cause ulcers. Sometimes it's difficult to know what causes an ulcer such as vascular disease, cancer, or scleroderma.

ACTION

To help heal a superficial ulcer you need a drawing agent to pull the dead cells out. If you know the underlying cause, treat that as well, for example an infection. Use one of the suggested remedies. If there is visible bleeding, see the section on "Bleeding" for additional help. Also see "Bed Sores."

KITCHEN REMEDIES

Honey–Take 1 teaspoon 1-2 times daily, if not a diabetic, and spread some over the skin ulcer.

Sage–Use this for indurated and various skin sores as it is an antiseptic and soothes ulcer. Take as a tea and use as a poultice.

Aloe Vera Plant–Cut a small piece of this natural antibiotic and pain relieving plant and apply directly to the skin ulcer several times daily, or slicing the piece length wise and bandage or scotch tape it to the area. You can use a fresh slice 1-2 times per day or overnight as needed.

Apple Cider Vinegar–Good to use to clean the skin around the ulcer.

SINGLE HERBAL REMEDIES

Burdock Root–To foment a skin ulcer apply warm liquid with a cloth or directly to the affected area. Keep moist by adding the liquid to the cloth or redampen cloth by immersion and reapply.

Chickweed–This is great for blood toxicity and inflammations Take as a tea and use as a fomentation.

Irish Moss–This remedy is soothing to the inflamed tissues. You can use Irish moss for external ulcers by applying the tea as a fomentation.

Marigold–A great first aid remedy that works particularly well for ulcers, and is very effective on old or badly healed scars. Use as an antiseptic tea and fomentation.

COMMERCIALLY PREPARED HERBAL REMEDIES

Herbs: Myrrh-Golden Seal Plus Formula (for ulcers and ulcerations); Ex-Stress Formula (Calms nervous system.); Kalmin (antispasmodic) (Nature's Way); Cabbage tablets; Ulfre (Helps ulcers and ulcerations) (Michael's); Rescue Remedy (for shock and trauma) (Bach); or, Liquid Trace Mineral (A great tissue healer that can be mixed with a 1/2 ounce of the mineral in 4-6 ounces of vegetable or fruit juice several times daily.).

Homeopathic: Nervousness; Emotional; Indigestion; Neuralgic Pains; Exhaustion; Emotional; or, Pain (Natra Bio); Indigestion & Gas; Menopause; or, PMS (Medicine From Nature).

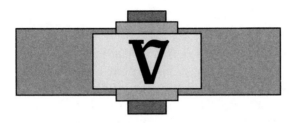

VAGINITIS

Vaginitis, a common problem for women, is a general term that means any infection or irritation of the vagina. Hormonal changes, such as during menopause, can also cause vaginitis. Symptoms may include vaginal irritation, itching, burning, soreness or tenderness, and sometimes a discharge with or without odor. Painful urination from urine irritating infected vulvar tissues can also be a sign. Dryness in the genital area may occur if the vaginitis is due to hormonal changes.

Some of the usual causes are yeast, bacterial, or protozoan (like Trichomonas) infections. Infections can be sexually transmitted particularly chlamydia, gonorrhea, or herpes. Excessive douching, feminine hygiene products, topical vaginal remedies and perfumed toilet paper can cause a chemical irritation in the genital region. Introduction of foreign objects into the vagina or sexual intercourse can damage the vaginal and surrounding tissue. If something becomes lodged in the vagina, it can produce a foul smell. Increased vaginal discharge, particularly when there is no abnormal smell or color, is a normal monthly event. This occurs in most women around the time of ovulation. Treatment is unnecessary in this situation.

If vaginitis is a recurring or chronic problem, have your doctor give you a diagnosis. Finding the cause is important so you can apply the correct remedy.

I highly recommend reading either one or both of the following books if you having a chronic problem with vaginitis due to a yeast infection, *The Yeast Connection* by Dr. Crook, M.D., or *The Missing Diagnosis* by C. O. Truss, M.D.

ACTION

If you are douching on a regular basis, stop. Douching disrupts the vagina's natural, healthy environment and encourages infections. You should of course wash the vaginal area with a natural soap and water, but not excessively. Use a natural disinfectant and keep it on for a few minutes before applying a remedy or mixing a suggested remedy with it.

Also, think about all the products that come into contact with your vagina: toilet paper, hygiene products, underwear, soap. Do you use a perfumed laundry detergent. Use plain, perfume-free, white toilet paper. Discontinue the use of all vaginal products. Switch to white, 100 percent cotton underpants. Don't wear underwear with your panty hose. Stop using spermicide creams, ointments, or gels and any other barrier contraceptive that contains spermicides. (In the meantime, use another form of birth control or abstain.)

If you discover you have a sexually transmitted disease, be sure to inform you partner(s) and have them treated as well. Refrain from sexual intercourse during treatment.

If you have a vaginal yeast infection, see "Yeast Infections" for dietary suggestions. In general, when you have an infection anywhere in the body, avoid sugar as it depresses your body's ability to fight infections.

KITCHEN REMEDIES

Apple Cider Vinegar–Fill a douche bulb or bag with water or an herbal tea (see "Herbal Remedies" below) and add 2 tablespoons of apple cider vinegar. You can use this solution as a douche or vaginal implant for 30 minutes.

Baking Soda–Use 1/4 teaspoon in douche water or do an implant to reduce acid burning feeling.

Sage–Use sage in a vaginal implant by adding 1/4-1/2 teaspoon to one pint of water. If the outer genital area is affected, treat it with a sage poultice.

Garlic–Mash, chop, or grate a clove of garlic, then blend in a cup of water or herbal tea. Drink 1/4 teaspoon of this liquid 3 times a day. Use a little of this solution in a vaginal implant. You can also apply this solution on the outer genital area, but first spread on some vegetable oil.

Yogurt–Use only unpasteurized or homemade yogurt as it is the best. Eat one cup of yogurt daily. Mix one pint of yogurt mixed with some water as a vaginal implant. You can also apply this mixture to the outer genital area if it's irritated. You can insert the yogurt with a tampon applicator. The culture in yogurt helps restore the natural bacterial flora of the vagina.

SINGLE HERBAL REMEDIES

Any of the herbs listed below may be taken as a tea for internal support or used as a vaginal implant. To do most implants add 20 drops of the selected herbal remedy to one pint of water. For some herbal implants, less plant is needed. See individual listings for instructions.

Black Walnut or Pau d'Arco–Either of these are great for vaginal infections. Take the tea and use as an implant.

Red Raspberry–The astringent actions of this herb are useful when there is an unusual vaginal discharge. You can use red raspberry in three ways: as an implant, tea, and applied directly on the irritated outer area.

Myrrh–This is great against bacteria and viruses. In the implant, use only 5 drops of myrrh. Make a tea and drink 2-3 times a day.

Echinacea–You may mix with red raspberry to boost this blood purifier and infection fighter. Make a tea and drink 2-3 times a day. Also, you can apply echinacea directly to the outer area of the genitals.

OTHER NATURAL TREATMENTS

Acidophilus–Take 2 capsules or 1 tablet 2-3 times daily for vaginal yeast infections. Also use for vaginal implants. You may use a tampon applicator soaked with acidophilus for an implant by dissolving 2 capsules in a total of 1 pint of water.

Douche: As many remedies in this section are applied exclusively or partially as douches, see "Kitchen Remedies" and "Herbal Remedies" for suggestions.

Vaginal Implants: Many of the remedies suggested for this section are used as vaginal implants. See above sections for suggestions.

COMMERCIALLY PREPARED HERBAL REMEDIES

Herbs: Yeast Fighters (for Candida Yeast) (Twin Labs); Rainbow; Cantrol and Caprinex (Nature's Way); Yeast Wafers (Standard Process); YeastGard suppositories (Women's Health Institute); Cal-Silica Formula (natural calcium); (Nature's Way); Calcium Citrate (Twin Lab); liquid trace mineral (Great for cleansing and healing and to use as a vaginal holding douche as needed. Also, take 1/2 ounce in about 4-6 ounces of vegetable or fruit juice several times daily.).

Homeopathic: Candida Yeast; Bladder Irritation; Neuralgic Pains; Menopause; Menstrual; Detoxification, Raw Female, Pain (Natra-Bio); Menopause; or Vaginitis (Medicine From Nature).

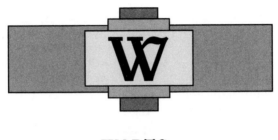

WARTS

Unsightly as warts are, they are usually harmless. The exception to this rule is venereal warts. These warts, left untreated, can lead to cancer.

However, in this chapter I'm going to focus on warts found on other parts of the body. Since warts are caused by viruses, they can be contagious and you can reinfect yourself if you are not attentive. Warts appear protruding from the skin, may be flat or long and narrow when on the face, neck, lips or eyelids. Plantar's warts, found on the sole of the foot, are flattened from the pressure of walking and standing. Warts can be rough or round, gray, yellow, or brown.

I have found that warts are usually due to poor nutrition and cleansing of the body eliminating channels, like the kidneys, and bowels. Poor immunity also encourages warts to grow. Most warts will spontaneously disappear in a few months with or without treatment. They do have a high recurrence rate and can reappear one-third of the time.

ACTION

Wash the wart with a natural soap and water. Then use a natural disinfectant. Improve your health and immunity by eating more vegetables, fruits, fibers and whole grains. Drink plenty of water and use one of the suggested remedies. You also need to pumice the dead skin over the wart at least 2 times a week with an emery board.

KITCHEN REMEDIES

Castor Oil–Works as a dissolver and cleanser. Spread directly over the wart using a piece of cotton taped to area.

Dandelion–Using this weed to treat warts is an old Asian folk remedy. The dandelion, a common garden weed, is rich in vitamins A, B complex, C, and many minerals such as potassium. It cleanses both the liver and skin. For several days apply the juice from a broken stem to warts and let it dry. Blend stems in with a little juice. You can also purchase dandelion ointment for direct application on the wart. You can make a tea of fresh dandelion leaves or use the dried herb, tincture, or capsules from the health food store. Drink 2-3 times a day.

> **WARNING:** Don't use dandelions from your yard if they've been sprayed with insecticides.

Garlic–You can slice a small sliver of fresh garlic and secure it with a bandage over the wart. But, first be sure to spread some vegetable oil over the wart so that the garlic won't irritate the skin. You can also apply garlic oil alone or mixed in with herbs directly over the wart. Also, make a tea by putting 5-8 drops of the oil or 1-2 capsules in a cup of hot or room temperature water, or in juice. Drink 2-3 times a day. Be persistent with this treatment. Garlic fights the wart virus.

Lemon–Fresh lemon is best to fight this viral infection. Squeeze some juice on a piece of cotton and tape it to the wart. Be persistent in the continuous use of this remedy, as it takes a while.

Meat Tenderizer–Mix the tenderizer, that works as an antiseptic, with a little castor or olive oil to make enough paste to cover the wart and cover with a bandage.

Onions, Kelp, or Seaweed–Add any of these edibles in quantity to the foods you are eating. They are all highly nutritious. Onions, like garlic, is a natural anti-viral remedy.

Pineapple–You can slice a small sliver of fresh pineapple and secure it to the wart with a bandage. Or, you can make poultice. As with the lemon, be persistent in applying this remedy that works as a cleanser. Bromelain, found in pineapple, is an enzyme that may help eliminate warts.

Papaya–Contains the enzyme, papain, that breaks down protein and dissolves warts. Use the fresh papaya as a poultice or spread the papaya juice over the area and cover with a piece of cotton or bandage.

Thyme–A powerful antiseptic that is good for any kind of infectious skin problem. Make a tea and drink 2-3 times a day. Also, you may apply warm thyme tea as a fomentation directly to the affected area. Keep moist by adding the liquid to the cloth or redampen cloth by immersion and reapply. For a stronger herbal effect, you can purchase thyme as a tincture or other extract from the health food store.

SINGLE HERBAL REMEDIES

Pau d'Arco–This Brazilian tree kills viruses. Apply a pau d'arco fomentation directly to the wart. You can also make a tea from this herb.

Jojoba Oil–Works as a strong cleanser. Apply directly to the wart, covering with a bandage or a taped piece of cotton.

Sassafras Oil–This is another strong cleanser that can be applied directly to the wart. After the oil dries, you can also use an emery board or pumice stone daily to buff off dead skin.

Wintergreen Oil–Works as a great antiseptic when applied directly to the wart. Cover with a bandage if necessary.

OTHER NATURAL TREATMENTS

Vitamin E (200 IU)–Dissolves the wart. Take direct 1-2 capsules per day and apply by puncturing the perle and squeezing the contents out to spread on the outer area.

COMMERCIALLY PREPARED HERBAL REMEDIES

Herbs: Red Clover Combination (Purifies blood stream); PARA-X (Cleanses parasites and toxic waste matter.); Liveron (Cleanses the liver and gall bladder) (Nature's Way).

Homeopathic: Thuja Occidentalis; or, Detoxification (Natra Bio).

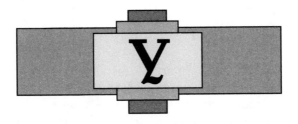

YEAST INFECTIONS

Yeast is found in virtually everybody. Under normal conditions, yeast does not cause any troubles. Usually yeast resides in harmony with friendly bacteria in our gut and other systems. When this balance is upset, an overgrowth occurs somewhere in the body and you have a fungal infection (yeast is a fungus). Events that kill off the friendly bacteria such as antibiotics, feed yeast like sugars and fungus (like mushrooms), and lifestyle factors which suppress your immunity like IV drug use all increase your likelihood of developing a yeast infection. Other risk factors include the birth control pill, steroids, diabetes and pregnancy.

Candida albicans is the yeast usually responsible for yeast infections. These infections may be acute and short lived, such as some vaginal yeast infections, or they may be chronic and more long-term. These cases are referred to as yeast syndrome or chronic candidiasis. Symptoms differ depending on the location of the yeast infection.

When yeast infects the mouth and/or throat it's called thrush, a condition that sometimes strikes babies. Signs are usually white spots on the inside of the mouth, tongue, or throat accompanied by a lot of pain. Diaper rash can also be caused by yeast. Vaginitis is often due to yeast with itching and a white or yellow discharge. The birth control pill and pregnancy are frequent causes. Women can pass this infection onto their sexual partners. There are many other sites for a yeast infection to develop, but an ailment that's becoming more frequent and recognized is gastrointestinal (GI) candida or yeast infection. Often women with vaginal yeast infections, also have GI infections as well. In these cases, treat yourself for both vaginal and GI yeast.

ACTION

Eliminate all simple carbohydrate foods, like white flour, all sugars (including honey, brown sugar and fruit juices), yeast and yeast products and foods containing a lot of yeast or molds such as alcohol, dried fruits, cheeses, peanuts, and melons. Drink plenty of water to keep your bowels open, avoid citrus juices, and take in more complex carbohydrates. However, limit how many starchy vegetables you eat like parsnips, yams, potatoes, and corn.

For babies who are not nursing exclusively, give goat, whey, or nut milk and mashed, steamed vegetables. Dispense Caprylic Acid (an extract from the coconut) that you can obtain from a health store to kill yeast and use the other remedies listed. Don't add any sweeteners to herbal teas and other remedies. Avoid adding remedies to fruit juices.

KITCHEN REMEDIES

Sage–Make this toxin fighting and soothing tea. You can also add to each cup 1/4 teaspoon of cinnamon with a pinch of each of ginger and cayenne.

Yogurt–This remedy replaces the natural bacterial flora in your intestine and thus, displacing the overgrowth of yeast. Use this until you can get a stronger remedy such as acidophilus. Eat 1 cup daily. If you have a vaginal yeast infection, you can also douche with yogurt.

Buttermilk–A great antiseptic that is taken 3 times a day. Give 1 tablespoon and let it trickle down the throat if you have thrush to coat the passage way.

Garlic–Garlic, a natural antifungal medicine, is especially effective against Candida. Use freely in cooking. If you have garlic oil, give 2-5 drops of this antiseptic oil to a baby and about 10-15 drops for adults in vegetable juice 3-4 times daily.

SINGLE HERBAL REMEDIES

Red Raspberry–Raspberry's astringent properties soothes the pain of thrush. Make a tea and drink 2-3 times a day. Give the tea to babies in a baby bottle.

White Oak Bark–In addition to taking this antiseptic remedy as a tea, you can use it as a gargle throughout the day for a sore and infected throat. Make a tea by putting 15-25 drops of the liquid or 2 capsules in a cup of warm water, herbal tea, or in natural milk. Drink 3 times a day. Give 5-10 drops for babies and young children.

Echinacea–This is good for any infection and boosts the immune system. Make a tea and drink 2-3 times a day.

OTHER NATURAL TREATMENTS

Acidophilus–Lactobacillus acidophilus is a friendly bacteria found in the human gut. It is one of the bacterias that gets pushed out of the intestinal tract during a yeast overgrowth. Liquid is the best. Give 1/2 teaspoon in 2-3 ounce bottle of liquid for babies or 2 capsules or 1 tablespoon for adults 3 times daily. You can also insert an acidophilus capsule into the vagina like a suppository for vaginal yeast infections. Most acidophilus is milk-based. If you are lactose intolerant or allergic to milk, use the milk-free acidophilus.

COMMERCIALLY PREPARED HERBAL REMEDIES

Herbs: Caprylic Acid capsules or extract (Dissolve the contents of 1 opened capsule in a cup of warm water, natural milk or herbal tea. Give half of it in the morning and the other half in the evening in a regular warm baby's formula. Or, give 5-10 drops of the extract in juice or formula 1-2 times a day. If breast feeding give 1 capsule to the mother once a day.); Yeast Fighter (Has 6-8 supports) (Twin Labs); Rainbow; Cantrol and Caprinex; or, Liveron (Cleanses liver & Gall Bladder) (Nature's Way).

Homeopathic: Candid Yeast; Neuralgic Pains; Insomnia; or, Pain (Natra Bio); Insomnia; or, Vaginitis (Medicine From Nature); or, YeastGard (vaginal suppository) (Women's Health Institute).

GLOSSARY

Throughout this book there may be terminology that is not familiar to you, so I have included this section to give you a better understanding of the terms used.

Decoction: A type of tea made from the hard and woody parts of a plant, such as the bark, inner bark or roots. You must boil and steep this kind of tea longer than an infusion in order to remove the active ingredients from the herb.

Douche: A warm solution of water, liquid herbs, or other natural fluid substance directed into the vagina for cleansing and healing purposes.

Enemas: Water and/or solutions introduced into the rectum and colon for healing and cleansing purposes.

Enema, Releasing: This type of enema is used to simply flush the heavy toxins from the system quickly as possible.

Extract: The essence of the herb that is extracted by boiling it in water in a closed container to release the active ingredients from the bulk or pulpy herb.

Fasting: To refrain from eating solid foods for therapeutic reasons. The main purpose of fasting is to help clean the body of years of accumulated toxic wastes and to let the body rest. Fasts can be conducted with just water, or by drinking water and nutritious fluids such as juices and broths.

Fomentation: Strictly speaking a fomentation is an extremely hot moist compress placed on the body. When I refer to fomentations in this book, I'm talking about the essence of the herb, usually in liquid or oil form, applied by cloth or directly to the affected area.

Infusion: A tea made by adding boiling water to an herb and allowing it to steep. This process extracts the therapeutic, water soluble agents of the herb.

Implant: An herbal solution directed into a body orifice and held there to maximize its healing effects. **Rectal** implants are like mini-enemas, and are introduced into the anus. **Vaginal** implants are squeezed into the vagina.

Naturopathy: A body of medical knowledge drawn from nutrition, herbal medicines, homeopathy, physical medicine, exercise therapy, counseling, accupuncture, natural childbirth, and hydrotherapy.

Poultice: A paste made of chopped, grated, or powdered vegetables, fruits, or herbs, and a liquid such as water or oil. This mixture is applied directly to an injured or diseased part of the body for healing purposes.

Slant Board: An inclined board for lying on which administering a treatment. Typically, the head is placed at the lower end of the slant board and the feet at the high end.

Soak Bath: A warm to hot therapeutic bath used for relaxing, detoxification and healing purposes. The bath may contain herbs, Epsom salt, baking soda, or other substances to enhance its effects. Other times, the bath may just contain water.

Tinctures: An herbal solution where the essence of the herb is extracted into liquid concentrate by alcohol, glycerine or vinegar. These are used because water alone will not extract some of the essential properties and preserve the essences.

REMEDY FINDER

Study this chart and plan ahead, before an emergency. The left column lists the ailments, the right hand column gives a quick remedy list for the ailments. The best remedy is listed **first**. Remedy aid from foods and spices appear first, next are single herbs and combinations of herbs followed by homeopathics.

Vegetables or herbs can be used **internally** and/or **externally**, also in **liquid** and/or **poultice** form. Use the remedy you already have in your kitchen. Space does not allow for all possibilities to be listed; however, there are more options available in the individual entries.

There are many good herbal companies producing single or combination herbal remedies and homeopathics. Naturally, not all can be mentioned here. I refer to the more widely known manufacturers, but ask your local health food store which ones are available in your area. The main companies I refer to are Twin Lab, Nature's Way, Medicine from Nature, Natra-Bio, and BHI (Biological Homeopathic Industries).

The product Liquid Trace Minerals is made up of the trace minerals found in the old sea bed in Utah. It is bottled by many companies. Ask your health store for the name brand in your area.

Find the remedy you have on hand, then read the chapter pertaining to the problem for instructions on how to administer the herbal remedy.

PROBLEMS AND REMEDIES

Abscess   **Kitchen Remedies:** Cayenne, aloe vera, raisins, garlic, olive or castor oils, or Epsom salt.

Single Herbal Remedies: Goldenseal, sage, echinacea, black walnut extract, or myrrh.

Commercially Prepared Remedies: Kalmin, Cal-Silica, BF&C capsules and/or ointment, or, liquid trace minerals.

Homeopathics: Injuries, Headache & Pain, or, Teeth & Gums.

Allergies

Kitchen Remedies: Brewer's yeast, onions, thyme, salt water, or, horseradish.

Single Herbal Remedies: Bayberry, eucalyptus oil, lungwort, fenugreek, or garlic oil.

Commercially Prepared Remedies: HAS, Breathe-Aid, Kalmin, Allergy Care, BronCare, or Sinustop.

Homeopathics: Allergy, Hayfever, Sinus, Raw Lung, or Sinusitis.

Anxiety or Phobia

Kitchen Remedies: Raisins, hard candy, fruits, celery, or, sage.

Single Herbal Remedies: Valerian, cayenne, chamomile, hawthorn, or skullcap.

Commercially Prepared Remedies: PC Formula, Kalmin, Adren-Aid, Ex-stress, or Rescue Remedy.

Homeopathics: Raw Pancreas, Raw Adrenal, Raw Female or Male, Nervousness, PMS, Emotional, or Menopause.

Asthma

Kitchen Remedies: Garlic, onion, horseradish, sage, or ginger.

Single Herbal Remedies: Eucalyptus, mullein, fenugreek, pleurisy root, or elecampane.

Commercially Prepared Remedies: HAS, Comfrey-Mullein-Garlic Syrup, Breathe-Aid, Kalmin, Rescue Remedy, or Fenu-Thyme.

Homeopathics: Allergy, Sinus, Emotion, Laxative, Candida Yeast, or Raw Lung.

Backache

Kitchen Remedies: Castor and olive oil, cranberry juice (not blended with another fruit), parsley, prunes, or vitamin E.

Single Herbal Remedies: Queen of the Meadow, chaparral, or juniper berries.

Commercially Prepared Remedies: Kalmin, BF&C capsules and ointment, KB, Ex-Stress, Vegetable Calcium, or Naturalax 2.

Homeopathics: Raw Kidney, Neuralgic Pains, Injuries, Laxative, or Emotional.

Bedsores

Kitchen Remedies: Aloe vera, apple cider vinegar, corn starch, castor, olive or wheat germ oils.

Single Herbal Remedies: Vitamin A, black walnut, myrrh, pau d'arco, or red clover.

Commercially Prepared Remedies: Chickweed ointments, BF&C capsules and ointment, AKN Skincare, Echinacea Combination, Myrrh-Goldenseal Plus, or liquid trace minerals.

Homeopathics: Silica, Injuries, Fever, Neuralgic Pains, Detoxification, or Candida Yeast.

Bites or Stings

Kitchen Remedies: Aloe vera, apple cider vinegar, meat tenderizer, lemon, or basil.

Single Herbal Remedies: Burdock, echinacea, skullcap, valerian root, or white oak bark.

Commercially Prepared Remedies: BF&C
capsules and ointment, Kalmin, Red Clover
Combination, Rescue Remedy, or liquid
trace minerals.

Homeopathics: Insect Bites, Injuries,
Detoxification, or SSSSTING Stop Ointment
(Boericke & Tafel).

Bleeding or Wounds **Kitchen Remedies:** Cayenne, sage, onion,
cranberry, or Witch Hazel.

Single Herbal Remedies: Alfalfa, aloe vera,
shepherd's purse, or white oak bark.

Commercially Prepared Remedies: BF&C
ointment and capsules, Myrrh-Goldenseal
Plus, Rescue Remedy, or liquid trace minerals.

Homeopathics: Injuries, Hemorrhoids,
Menstrual, or Bleeding.

Blisters   **Kitchen Remedies:** Corn starch, honey, apple
cider vinegar, wheat germ, and olive oils.

Single Herbal Remedies: Dandelion, aloe
vera, comfrey, or chickweed.

Commercially Prepared Remedies: BF&C,
Chickweed or Comfrey ointments, Pau d'arco
bark, Echinacea-Goldenseal Root
Combination, or liquid trace minerals.

Homeopathics: Injuries, Fever, or Pain.

Blood Poisoning   **Kitchen Remedies:** Cayenne, apple cider
vinegar, garlic, onion, or raisins.

Single Herbal Remedies: Echinacea, goldenseal, plantain, marshmallow, or red clover.

Commercially Prepared Remedies: Kalmin, H Formula, Red Clover Combination, or liquid trace minerals.

Homeopathics: Lachesis, Injuries, Fever, Pain, Nausea, or Detoxification.

Boils

Kitchen Remedies: Aloe vera, apple cider vinegar, garlic, onion, figs, raisins, or sage.

Single Herbal Remedies: burdock root, echinacea, red clover, sarsaparilla, or sassafras.

Commercially Prepared Remedies: BF&C, Chickweed and/or Black ointments, AKN Skincare, or Myrrh-Goldenseal Plus.

Homeopathics: Detoxification, Injuries, or Raw Liver.

Bones, broken

Kitchen Remedies: Aloe vera, apple cider vinegar, cayenne, sage, or legumes.

Single Herbal Remedies: Horsetail grass, oat straw, queen of the meadow, or skullcap.

Commercially Prepared Remedies: BF&C capsules and ointment, Cal-Silica, Bone All, Calcium Citrate, Rescue Remedy, or liquid trace minerals.

Homeopathics: Injuries, Neuralgic Pains, Emotional, or Pain.

Bruises

Kitchen Remedies: Aloe vera, castor, wheat germ and olive oils, safflower oil, or corn starch.

Single Herbal Remedies: Echinacea, marigold, St. John's wort, or bayberry.

Commercially Prepared Remedies: BF&C
ointment, Cal-Silica, Rescue Remedy, or liquid
trace minerals.

Homeopathics: Injuries, Pain, Calendula,
Hypericum, or Emotional.

Burns   **Kitchen Remedies:** Aloe vera, apple cider vinegar, honey, olive oil, witch hazel, or potato.

Single Herbal Remedies: Marigold, St. John's
wort, or vitamins A and E.

Commercially Prepared Remedies: BF&C,
Comfrey and Mullein ointments, Rescue
Remedy, or liquid trace minerals.

Homeopathics: Injuries, Pain, Insomnia,
Headache, or Cantharis 30-200X.

Chicken Pox,   **Kitchen Remedies:** Aloe vera, apple cider
Shingles   vinegar, celery, sage, or witch hazel.

Single Herbal Remedies: Red raspberry, tansy.

Commercially Prepared Remedies: BF&C
ointment, Ex-Stress, Cal-Silica, Kalmin, or liquid trace minerals.

Homeopathics: Pain, Calendula or Hypericum.

Colds and Flu   **Kitchen Remedies:** Sage, cinnamon, garlic,
lemon, ginger, horseradish, or apple cider vine-
gar.

Single Herbal Remedies: Echinacea, elder
flower, eucalyptus oil, peppermint, pleurisy
root, red raspberry, 50 mg. of vitamin B-6.

Commercially Prepared Remedies: Fenu-Thyme, GL Formula, HAS, Comfrey-M, Mullein-Garlic Syrup, or Winter Care Formula, Breathe Aide, Immunaid.

Homeopathics: Cold, Cough, Flu. Fever, Sore Throat, or Exhaustion.

Colic

Kitchen Remedies: Sage, apple cider vinegar, castor oil, olive oil, baking soda, lemon, or aloe vera, ginger.

Single Herbal Remedies: Catnip, fennel, wild yam, chamomile, valerian root, peppermint, or spearmint.

Commercially Prepared Remedies: Kalmin, Kol-X, Ex-Stress, or Calcium Citrate.

Homeopathics: Laxative, Teething, Indigestion & Gas, Calms, or Colic.

Constipation

Kitchen Remedies: Prunes, figs, aloe vera, sage, lemon, or olive oil.

Single Herbal Remedies: Dandelion, chaparral, senna leaves, or turkey rhubarb extract.

Commercially Prepared Remedies: Naturalax 2, Aloelax, Liveron, Ex-Stress, or Children's Fletcher's Castoria (unflavored).

Homeopathics: Laxative, Detoxification, Colic, Constipation and Hemorrhoids, or Indigestion & Gas.

Convulsions

Kitchen Remedies: Cayenne or honey.

Single Herbal Remedies: Valerian root, catnip, red clover, chamomile, passion flower, or peppermint.

Commercially Prepared Remedies: Kalmin, PC Formula, Ex-Stress, or Rescue Remedy.

Homeopathics: Emotional, Nervousness, Exhaustion, Raw Adrenal, or Raw Pancreas.

Coughing

Kitchen Remedies: Lemon and honey, apple cider vinegar, garlic, sage, or horseradish.

Single Herbal Remedies: Catnip, comfrey, cayenne, garlic oil, elder flower, fenugreek, mullein, or pleurisy root.

Commercially Prepared Remedies: HAS, Breathe-Aid Formula, Mullein-Garlic Syrup, Immunaid, or Herbal Influence Formula.

Homeopathics: Cough, Fever, Sinus, Cold and Flu, or Detoxification.

Depression

Kitchen Remedies: Catnip, chamomile, sage, honey, or raisins.

Single Herbal Remedies: Red raspberry, St. John's wort, or wormwood, Valerian root.

Commercially Prepared Remedies: PC Formula, Silent Night, Calcium Citrate, Rescue Remedy, or Cal-Silica.

Homeopathics: Nervousness, Exhaustion, Fatigue, PMS, Menstrual, or Emotional.

Diarrhea

Kitchen Remedies: Allspice, sage, barley water, apple cider vinegar, cloves, activated charcoal, cinnamon, or peppermint.

Single Herbal Remedies: Bayberry, catnip, myrrh, or comfrey root.

Commercially Prepared Remedies: Kalmin, Ex-Stress, Cal-Silica, Rescue Remedy, or liquid trace minerals.

Homeopathics: Diarrhea, Colic, Nausea, or Teething.

Dizziness

Kitchen Remedies: Grape juice, honey, apples, sage, cloves, garlic, or raisins.

Single Herbal Remedies: Lemon grass, catnip, rose hips, chamomile, valerian root, or skull-cap.

Commercially Prepared Remedies: PC Formula, Adren-Aid, Motion Mate, Change-O-Life, or Rescue Remedy.

Homeopathics: Nausea, Tension, Emotional, or PMS.

Ear

Kitchen Remedies: Garlic, olive oil, apple cider vinegar, sage, or cabbage.

Single Herbal Remedies: Mullein, echinacea, cloves, Pau d'arco, or glycerine.

Commercially Prepared Remedies: Kalmin, B&B Formula, GL Formula, or liquid trace minerals.

Homeopathics: Earache, Fever, Sinus, or Cold and Flu.

Exhaustion   **Kitchen Remedies:** Sage, almond nut milk, juices, powerhouse drink.

Single Herbal Remedies: Sarsaparilla, echinacea, or Siberian ginseng.

Commercially Prepared Remedies: Adren-Aid, PC Formula, Cal-Silica, H Formula, Ex-Stress, or liquid trace minerals.

Homeopathics: Exhaustion, Insomnia, Fatigue, Emotional, or Detoxification.

Eyes   **Kitchen Remedies:** Aloe vera, castor oil, cod liver oil, onions, witch hazel, or eggs.

Single Herbal Remedies: Eyebright, burdock, echinacea, mullein, sassafras, or goldenseal.

Commercially Prepared Remedies: Eyebright Combination, liquid trace minerals, Ex-Stress, or Rescue Remedy.

Homeopathics: Eye Irritation, Injuries, Pain, or Headache.

Fainting   **Kitchen Remedies:** Cayenne, honey, raisins, grapes, apple cider vinegar, peppermint, or spearmint.

Single Herbal Remedies: Chamomile, catnip, valerian root, or lemon grass.

Commercially Prepared Remedies: Kalmin, Adren-Aid, PC Formula, or Ex-Stress, or liquid trace minerals.

Homeopathics: Raw Adrenal, Raw Pancreas, Emotional, Injuries, or Fatigue.

Fever

Kitchen Remedies: Cloves, garlic, apple cider vinegar, barley water, lemon juice, or ginger.

Single Herbal Remedies: Echinacea, red raspberry, lemon grass, or feverfew.

Commercially Prepared Remedies: GL Formula, Fenu-Thyme, Breathe-Aid, Winter Care Formula, or Kalmin.

Homeopathics: Fever, Flu, Teething, Earache, or Colds and Flu.

Food Poisoning

Kitchen Remedies: Sage, spearmint tea, ginger, baking soda, activated charcoal, apple cider vinegar, carbonated water, blessed thistle, or salt.

Single Herbal Remedies: Red Raspberry, sarsaparilla, sassafras, fennel, gentian, or burdock root.

Commercially Prepared Remedies: Kalmin, Naturalax 1, 2, or 3, Aloelax, or Liveron.

Homeopathics: Nausea, Headache and pain, Indigestion, Laxative, Colic, Diarrhea.

Frostbite

Kitchen Remedies: Aloe vera, olive or wheat germ oils, cayenne, or cinnamon.

Single Herbal Remedies: Vitamins A and/or E, echinacea, or Siberian ginseng.

Commercially Prepared Remedies: Rescue Remedy, Adren-Aid, Immunaid, or Winter Care Formula.

Homeopathics: Injuries, Emotional, Cold and Flu, Earache, or Cold

Fungus

Kitchen Remedies: Aloe vera, garlic, onion, lemon, figs, wheat germ, castor oils, or corn starch.

Single Herbal Remedies: Black walnut extract, chickweed, Pau d'arco, or myrrh.

Commercially Prepared Remedies: BF&C capsules and ointment, liquid trace minerals, Red Clover Combination, Para-X, or Para-VF Syrup.

Homeopathics: Mycosode, Mycological Immune Stimulator (Professional Health Products), or Candida yeast.

Gall Stones

Kitchen Remedies: Apple juice, sage, or parsley.

Single Herbal Remedies: Dandelion, barberry, fennel, or wild yam.

Commercially Prepared Remedies: Liveron, Kalmin, Cal-Silica, liquid trace minerals, or Rescue Remedy.

Homeopathics: Gallbladder, Nausea, Pain, or Indigestion & Gas.

Gout

Kitchen Remedies: Sage, apple cider vinegar, celery, parsley, castor, or olive oil.

Single Herbal Remedies: Burdock root, dandelion, devil's claw, or queen of the meadow.

Commercially Prepared Remedies: BF&C capsules and ointment, Liveron, Rheum-Aid, Cal-Silica, KB Formula, or liquid trace minerals.

Homeopathics: Raw Liver, Raw Kidney, Arthritis, Neuralgic Pains, or Detoxification.

Hangover   **Kitchen Remedies:** Black coffee, sage, or cayenne.

Single Herbal Remedies: Valerian, skullcap, or white willow bark.

Commercially Prepared Remedies: Adren-Aid, PC Formula, Liveron, Energizer Formula, or Calcium Citrate.

Homeopathics: Headache and Pain, Nausea, Nervousness, Detoxification, or Fatigue.

Headaches   **Kitchen Remedies**: Celery, onion, sage, apple cider vinegar, cayenne, or ginger.

Single Herbal Remedies: Black cohosh, chamomile, feverfew, passion flower, peppermint, or white willow.

Commercially Prepared Remedies: Kalmin, B/P Formula, CapsiCool, Ex-stress, liquid trace minerals.

Homeopathics: Headache and pain; injuries; Detoxification; Menstrual; Cold; Aches; or tension headaches.

Hemorrhoids or Anus **Kitchen Remedies:** Aloe vera plant, cayenne, sage, garlic, witch hazel, or cranberry.

Single Herbal Remedies: Red raspberry, tormentil root, marshmallow, or pau d'arco.

Commercially Prepared Remedies: BF&C capsules and ointment, Red Clover Combination, or liquid trace minerals.

Homeopathics: Hemorrhoids, Emotional, Varicose Veins, Pain, or Detoxification.

Hiccups

Kitchen Remedies: Apple cider vinegar, cayenne, sage, onion, or baking soda.

Single Herbal Remedies: Catnip, chamomile, wild lettuce, passion flower, or valerian root.

Commercially Prepared Remedies: Kalmin, Ex-Stress, Rescue Remedy;

Homeopathics: Emotional, Indigestion & Gas, Nervousness, or Injuries.

Hoarseness or
Laryngitis

Kitchen Remedies: Sage, garlic, lemon and honey, or salt.

Single Herbal Remedies: Echinacea, fenugreek, thyme, mullein, or lungwort.

Commercially Prepared Remedies: Kalmin, Ex-Stress, GL Formula, IF Formula, or Fenu-Thyme.

Homeopathics: Cough, Sinus, Earache, Cold and Flu, or Detoxification.

Indigestion

Kitchen Remedies: Baking soda, ginger, sage, peppermint, cloves, blessed thistle, potato, soft drink, garlic oil, or parsley.

Single Herbal Remedies: Chamomile, skullcap, or wild yam.

Commercially Prepared Remedies: Kalmin, Ex-stress, Naturalax 2, or Aloelax.

Homeopathics: Indigestion, laxative, colic, Emotional, or candida yeast.

Insect Repellent **Kitchen Remedies:** Apple cider vinegar, garlic, onion, wheat germ oil, or olive oil.

Single Herbal Remedies: Brewer's yeast, eucalyptus oil, penny royal, or repellent mixture.

Commercially Prepared Remedies: BF&C ointment, Kalmin, AKN Skincare, or Pau d'arco extract.

Homeopathics: Insect Bites, Detoxification, or SSSSting Stop.

Insomnia **Kitchen Remedies:** Sage, peppermint, spearmint, catnip, or milk (goat or soy).

Single Herbal Remedies: Blue vervain, chamomile, valerian root, lady's slipper, or passion flower.

Commercially Prepared Remedies: Kalmin, Silent Night, Ex-Stress, Rescue Remedy, or Sleepytime tea.

Homeopathics: Insomnia, Nervousness, Exhaustion, Emotional, or Fatigue.

Lice **Kitchen Remedies:** Aloe vera, garlic, onion, or apple cider vinegar.

Single Herbal Remedies: Black walnut extract, Pau d'arco extract, chaparral, echinacea, or thyme.

Commercially Prepared Remedies: Red Clover Combination, Para-X, Naturalax, Rescue Remedy, or liquid trace minerals.

Homeopathics: Insect Bites, Detoxification, or Hair and Scalp.

Menstrual   **Kitchen Remedies:** Sage, beet juice, carrot juice, or witch hazel.

Single Herbal Remedies: Black cohosh, cramp bark, chamomile, catnip, or dong quai.

Commercially Prepared Remedies: Fem-Mend Formula, Change-O-Life, Ex-Stress, or Ladies Only (Crystal Springs).

Homeopathics: Menstrual, Raw Female, or Vaginitis.

Miscarriage   **Kitchen Remedies:** Olive or wheat germ oil.

Single Herbal Remedies: False or true unicorn, valerian root, cramp bark, or wild yam.

Commercially Prepared Remedies: Red Raspberry Combination, or Kalmin, Ex-Stress.

Homeopathics: Injuries, Emotional, Pain, or Headache.

Motion Sickness   **Kitchen Remedies:** baking soda, sage, cloves, ginger, peppermint, or spearmint.

Single Herbal Remedies: Red raspberry or ginger root.

Commercially Prepared Remedies: Motion Mate, Adren-Aid, PC Formula, Ex-Stress, or Liveron.

Homeopathics: Nausea, Emotional, Detoxification, or Exhaustion.

Mumps   **Kitchen Remedies:** Cayenne, sage, corn flower, garlic, or onion.

Single Herbal Remedies: Red raspberry, myrrh, fenugreek, echinacea, or boneset.

Commercially Prepared Remedies: GL Formula, Fenu-Thyme, Ex-Stress, or liquid trace minerals.

Homeopathics: Fever, Detoxification, Earache, Headache and Pain, or Raw Thymus.

Muscle Cramps   **Kitchen Remedies:** Catnip, peppermint, spearmint, castor, olive, or wheat germ oils.

Single Herbal Remedies: Chamomile, valerian root, black cohosh, cramp bark, or myrrh extract.

Commercially Prepared Remedies: Kalmin, Cal-Silica, Ex-Stress, Rescue Remedy, or liquid trace minerals.

Homeopathics: Injuries, Aches and Pains, or Fatigue.

Nausea or Vomiting   **Kitchen Remedies:** Basil, sage. baking soda, apple cider vinegar, or cayenne.

Single Herbal Remedies: Red raspberry, peppermint, spearmint, or valerian root.

Commercially Prepared Remedies: Kalmin, Motion Mate, or Rescue Remedy.

Homeopathics: Nausea, Detoxification, Emotional, or Colic.

Nightmares   **Kitchen Remedies:** Sage, thyme, or marjoram.

Single Herbal Remedies: Catnip, peppermint, spearmint, or skullcap.

Commercially Prepared Remedies: Cal-Silica, Kalmin, Ex-Stress, Silent Night, or Rescue Remedy.

Homeopathics: Insomnia, Indigestion & Gas, Menopause, Emotional, or Detoxification.

Poisons   *Follow the directions on the label of any ingested poisons.*

Prostate   **Kitchen Remedies:** Sage, cranberry juice, parsley, castor oil, or olive oil.

Single Herbal Remedies: Burdock root, buchu, or saw palmetto.

Commercially Prepared Remedies: Kalmin, Red Clover Combination, Cal-Silica, ExStress, or PR Formula.

Homeopathics: Prostate, Raw Male, Detoxification, or Injury.

Rashes   **Kitchen Remedies:** Sage, meat tenderizer, baking soda, aloe vera, or apple cider vinegar.

Single Herbal Remedies: Plantain, black walnut extract, burdock root, or chickweed.

Commercially Prepared Remedies: Kalmin, AKN Skincare, Ex-Stress, or liquid trace minerals.

Homeopathics: Nervousness, Poison Oak, Poison Ivy, Detoxification, or Candida Yeast.

Sciatica

Kitchen Remedies: Apple cider vinegar, wheat germ oil, cayenne, or garlic.

Single Herbal Remedies: Peppermint oil, sassafras oil, rosemary oil, or thyme oil.

Commercially Prepared Remedies: Cal-Silica, BF&C capsules and ointment, Kalmin, Calcium Citrate, or Naturalax 2.

Homeopathics: Sciatica, Neuralgic Pains, Emotional, Detoxification, or Injury and Backache.

Sinusitis

Kitchen Remedies: Sage, salt, garlic, or onion.

Single Herbal Remedies: Mullein, peppermint oil, eucalyptus oil, or fennel.

Commercially Prepared Remedies: HAS, Breathe-Aid, Echinacea Combination, Fenu-Thyme, or Sinustop.

Homeopathics: Cold and Flu, Fever, Earache, Allergy, or Sinusitis.

Splinters

Kitchen Remedies: Aloe vera, apple cider vinegar, cayenne, meat tenderizer, or sage.

Single Herbal Remedies: Wood betony, southern wood, agrimony, or hawthorn.

Commercially Prepared Remedies: Echinacea Combination, BF&C ointment, Black Ointment, or liquid trace minerals.

Homeopathics: Injuries, Insect Bites, or Pain.

Sprains

Kitchen Remedies: Pressure held directly on the sprained area when possible, sage, apple cider vinegar, or olive oil.

Single Herbal Remedies: Wintergreen oil, catnip, or burdock.

Commercially Prepared Remedies: BF&C ointment, Cal-Silica, Ex-Stress, Liquid Trace Minerals, or Rescue Remedy.

Homeopathics: Injuries, or Pain.

Strep Throat

Kitchen Remedies: Buttermilk, yogurt, garlic, onion, or sage.

Single Herbal Remedies: Pau d'arco, echinacea, or garlic oil.

Commercially Prepared Remedies: Liquid trace minerals, Kalmin, Ex-Stress, or IF Formula.

Homeopathics: Laxative, Detoxification, or Sore Throat.

Sty

Kitchen Remedies: Aloe vera, hot/cold packs, onion, sage, or olive oil.

Single Herbal Remedies: Burdock root, red raspberry, marshmallow, fennel, or myrrh.

Commercially Prepared Remedies: Eyebright, Eyebright Combination, Liveron, Cal-Silica, or liquid trace minerals.

Homeopathics: Eye Irritation or Cold Sores/Fever Blisters.

Sunburn

Kitchen Remedies: Aloe vera, sage, apple cider vinegar, Witch Hazel, or honey.

Single Herbal Remedies: Bayberry, calendula, vitamin E.

Commercially Prepared Remedies: BF&C capsules and ointment, Silent Night, or liquid trace minerals.

Homeopathics: Injuries, Neuralgic Pains, Fever, Insomnia, or Headache.

Swollen Glands   **Kitchen Remedies:** Spiced sage tea, apple cider vinegar, castor oil, parsley, garlic, or horseradish.

Single Herbal Remedies: Thyme, mullein, echinacea, marshmallow, oak bark, bayberry, or goldenseal.

Commercially Prepared Remedies: GL Formula, IF Formula, Thyme, liquid trace minerals.

Homeopathics: Flue, Cold, Earache, Sore Throat, or Sinus.

Teething   **Kitchen Remedies:** Sage, cayenne, wheat germ oil.

Single Herbal Remedies: Fennel extract, clove oil, or red raspberry.

Commercially Prepared Remedies: Cal-Silica, BF&C capsules, Kalmin Extract, liquid calcium with vitamin D.

Homeopathics: Teething, Teeth and Gums, Neuralgic Pains, Detoxification, or Colic.

Teeth Grinding   **Kitchen Remedies:** Sage, catnip, chamomile, peppermint, or spearmint tea.

Single Herbal Remedies: Horsetail or oat straw.

Commercially Prepared Remedies: Calcium-Silica, Calcium Citrate, BF&C, or Kalmin.

Homeopathics: Calcium Carbonate 6-12x (see a homeopath).

Toenail, Ingrown   **Kitchen Remedies:** Aloe vera, apple cider vinegar, castor oil, olive oil, or wheat germ oil.

Single Herbal Remedies: Plantain or vitamins A and E.

Commercially Prepared Remedies: Cal-Silica, BF&C capsules and ointment, Vegetarian, Calcium, or liquid trace minerals.

Homeopathics: Injuries, Headache and Pain, Pain, or Detoxification.

Tonsils   **Kitchen Remedies:** Ginger or sage.

Single Herbal Remedies: Bayberry, black walnut extract, marshmallow, mullein, and red raspberry.

Commercially Prepared Remedies: GL Formula, IF Formula, Kalmin, Liveron, or liquid trace minerals.

Homeopathics: Fever, Sore Throat, Earache, Cold and Flu, or Headache and Pain.

Toothache   **Kitchen Remedies:** Cayenne, sage, apple cider vinegar, cloves, or ice pack.

Single Herbal Remedies: Clove oil, camphor oil, or sassafras oil.

Commercially Prepared Remedies: Kalmin, Cal-Silica, Echinacea Combination, Rescue Remedy, or liquid trace minerals.

Homeopathics: Toothache, Headache and Pain, Injuries, Neuralgic Pains, or Earache.

Traumatic Shock   **Kitchen Remedies:** Cayenne, sage, celery.

Single Herbal Remedies: Shock drink, catnip, red clover, mullein, or skullcap.

Commercially Prepared Remedies: Kalmin, Ex-stress, liquid trace minerals, or Rescue Remedy.

Homeopathics: Emotional, Injuries, Neuralgic Pains, or Nervousness.

Ulcers   **Kitchen Remedies:** Cayenne, aloe vera plant, cabbage, or baking soda.

Single Herbal Remedies: Burdock root, chick-weed, goldenseal, or Irish moss.

Commercially Prepared Remedies: Myrrh-Goldenseal Plus, Ex-Stress, Kalmin, cabbage tablets, or Ulfre (Michael's Products).

Homeopathics: Emotional, Indigestion and Gas, or Neuralgic Pains.

Ulcers, skin   **Kitchen Remedies**: Honey, sage, aloe vera plant, or apple cider vinegar.

Single Herbal Remedies: Burdock root, chick-weed, Irish moss, or marigold.

Commercially Prepared Remedies: Kalmin, Ex-stress, cabbage tablets, Ulfre, or Rescue Remedy.

Homeopathics: Nervousness, Emotional, Indigestion, Neuralgic Pains, or Exhaustion.

Vaginitis

Kitchen Remedies: Apple cider vinegar, baking soda, sage, or garlic.

Single Herbal Remedies: Acidophilus, black walnut, Pau d'arco, or red raspberry.

Commercially Prepared Remedies: Yeast Fighter, Cantrol (Rainbow), Yeast Wafers, Caprinex.

Homeopathics: Raw Female, Vaginitis, Candida Yeast, Menopause, or Menstrual.

Warts

Kitchen Remedies: Castor oil, dandelion weed juice, garlic, or lemon.

Single Herbal Remedies: Sassafras oil, Pau d'arco, or jojoba oil.

Commercially Prepared Remedies: Red Clover Combination, Para-X, or Liveron.

Homeopathics: Thuja Occidentalis (mother tincture) or Detoxification.

Yeast Infections

Kitchen Remedies: Sage, garlic, cayenne yogurt, or buttermilk.

Single Herbal Remedies: Red raspberry, echinacea, white oak bark, or acidophilus.

Commercially Prepared Remedies: Caprylic Acid, Yeast Fighters, Cantrol (Rainbow), Caprinex, or Liveron.

Homeopathic: Candida Yeast, Neuralgic Pains, Insomnia, Pain, Vaginitis, or YeastGard.

HERBAL HELPER

This chart gives you a match up between various remedies in the kitchen (single or in combination) and the problems they help to alleviate. Based on the needs of your family, you can make a natural remedy kit from these listings.

   This listing is a quick reference to jog your memory and help you be aware of the healing properties you have on hand. Not all the remedies listed in the individual entries are contained in this list, particularly if the remedy is only for one specific problem. I have found it helpful to keep more broad based remedies on hand unless you have a chronic condition. When you have selected a remedy refer to the entry on the problem for administration instructions.

KITCHEN REMEDIES

REMEDY	PROBLEM
Almond Oil	Stones and gravel, energy and nerve disorders, gall bladder ducts, or inflamed hands and skins.
Aloe Vera	Various cuts, bites, stings, sores, fungus, burns, constipation, and infections.
Apple Cider Vinegar	Antiseptic, cuts, burns boils, infections, bedsores, blisters, gas, colic, diarrhea, dizziness, bites, or stings.
Baking Soda	Bites, stings, indigestion, gas, or colic.
Basil	Cold, wet weather, nervous disorders, stomach disorders, or headaches.

Barley Water	Diarrhea or nausea.
Carrot, Potato, Tomato	Drawing and healing for painful bruises and infections.
Castor Oil	Congestion, hard nodules, warts, muscles, blisters, bruises, false labor pains, or colic.
Cayenne	Abscess, bleeding, cuts, heart problems, ulcers, infections, flu, colds, blood pressure, or toothache..
Celery Powder or Fresh	Diuretic, gas, neuralgic pains, headaches, sleeplessness, or stress. Feeds and calms the nervous system
Cinnamon	Diarrhea, nausea, frostbite, colds, flu, congestion, inflammation, indigestion, mild cardiac stimulator, and motion sickness.
Cloves	Toothaches, infections, gas, breath freshener, or nausea.
Cornflower (Yellow)	Mumps or food poisoning.
Corn Starch	Rashes, bed sores, bruises, or soreness.
Cranberry Juice	Diuretic, stops simple bleeding in urine.
Epsom Salt	Poisons, sprains, soreness, abscess, or blisters.
Fennel	Indigestion, colic, gas, bowels, gall bladder, and a mild laxative for babies and children.
Garlic	Infections, sores, boils, colds, flu, congestion, gas, sores, or ulcers.
Ginger	Gas, intestinal disorders, colic, feverish colds, flu, menstrual cycle, food poisoning, dysentery, congestion, inflammation.

Horseradish	Sinus, sore throat, glands, colds, congestions, asthma, coughing, and various infections.
Lemon	Colic, liver, gall bladder, stomach, bowels, colds, sore throat, congestion, antiseptic, bites and stings.
Mustard	Flu, cold, earaches, ulcerated tooth, sinusitis, pneumonia, or, inflammation. Great for body or foot baths.
Mayonnaise	Helps neutralize bites and various stings.
Meat Tenderizer	Neutralizes the acid in bites and stings.
Olive Oil	Gall bladder, bruises, muscles, bed sores, blisters, or colic.
Onion	Indigestion, sleeplessness, coughs, or sunburn.
Parsley	Colic, stomach disorders, kidney, bladder, eye infections, or general pain.
Sage	Food poisoning, diarrhea, nausea, colic, flu, fever, gas, sore throat, pain, headache, motion sickness, vaginitis, or teething.
Salt	Food poisoning, poisons, sore throat, sprains, bruises, or, skin ulcers.
Thyme	Nerves, sedative, ear infections, allergies, congestion, mucus, infections, antiseptic, and teeth.
Wheat Germ Oil	Bruises, infections, pain, soreness, bed sores, or rashes.
Witch Hazel	Bites, stings, cuts, infections, sores, and antiseptic.

SINGLE HERBAL REMEDIES

REMEDY   PROBLEM

Alfalfa   Alcoholism and narcotic addictions.

Bayberry   Astringent and antiseptic, mucus mem-
                                branes, congestion, wounds, colitis, dysen-
                                tery, adrenal glands, tonsillitis, and sore
                                throat.

Black Cohosh   Heart problems, or menstrual cramps.

Black Walnut Extract   Various infections, sores, abscess, boils, par-
                                asites, or fungus.

Boneset   High fevers, chills, aches and flu.

Buchu   Prostate problems and urinary tract.

Burdock Root   Antiseptic, bites, stings, rabid animals, and
                                various bites.

Carob Powder   Diarrhea and nausea.

Catnip   Nerves, convulsions, diarrhea, nausea, chil-
                                dren's chills and fever, gas, indigestion,
                                colic, or convulsions.

Chamomile   Gas, colic, nerves, convulsions, shock, trau-
                                ma, and mild sedative.

Chaparral   Backaches, tissue, bowels, bloodstream, and
                                chemical burns.

Charcoal   Diarrhea, absorbs poisons, or nausea.

Chickweed   Plaque in blood stream, antiseptic, infec-
                                tions, and blisters.

Clove Oil	High fevers, flu, colds, or toothache.
Cramp Bark	Menstrual or pregnancy cramps, and mumps.
Dandelion	Bowels, tonic, warts, or blisters.
Dong Quai	Menstrual cycle regulator.
Echinacea	Chemical burns, colds, flu, congestion and immune system, sore throat, bites, stings, various infections, antiseptic, abscesses, and boils.
Elderberry	Fever and inflammation.
Elder Flower	Congestion, flu, colds, coughing, or fevers.
Elecampane	Mucus, congestion, or chronic asthma.
Eucalyptus Oil	Decongestant, nasal passages, expectorant, colds, flu, or sinus.
Eye Bright	All types of eye problems.
False or True Unicorn	Miscarriages, convulsions, or menstrual cycle.
Fenugreek	Congestion and mucus.
Feverfew	All types of fevers.
Figwort	Strep throat, skin diseases, or fungus.
Fo-Ti-Ting	Hangover, brain and memory.
Goldenseal	Infections, bites, stings, cuts, and various wounds.
Hawthorn Berry	Heart, calms palpitations, miscarriage, or strokes.

Horsetail Grass   Bones and cartilage.

Juniper Berry   Infections, regulates blood sugar, mucus, lumbago, backache, and sciatica.

Irish Moss   Stomach (peptic) ulcers.

Lady's Slipper   Nervous system, pain, hiccups, and convulsions.

Lemon Grass   Fever, colds, flu, stress headaches, or fainting.

Licorice   Pancreas and blood sugar.

Lungwort   Expectorant, mucus, and hoarseness.

Marigold   Teeth, ear aches, bruises, burns, various injuries & wounds, nerve pain, old scarring ulcers, and various infections.

Marshmallow   Mucus, various infections, hemorrhoids, antiseptic, and various blood poisoning.

Mistletoe   Uterine contractions, bleeding, blood pressure, low adrenals, or hypertension.

Mullein   Mucus, lung congestion, bowels, cough, hayfever, or sinuses.

Myrrh   Chronic diarrhea, and various infections.

Oat Straw   Bones and teeth grinding.

Parsley Root   Jaundice, kidney stones, bladder inflammation, spleen obstructions, or indigestion.

Passion Flower   Convulsions, nerves, nervousness, insomnia, or mumps.

Pau d'arco   Various infections, parasites, bacteria, sores, abrasions, wounds, and boils.

Peppermint	Nerves, convulsions, appendicitis, chest, lungs, congestion, diarrhea, nausea, inflammation, flu, children's chills, fever, nerve relaxant, colic, convulsions various infections, and antiseptic.
Pleurisy Root	Cough, lung congestion, pleurisy, flu, or colds.
Queen of the Meadow	Joints, muscles, vertebrate pains, sprains, aches, kidney, stones, backache, or prostate.
Red Clover	Blood stream, blood infections, and normalizes RH factor of the blood.
Red Raspberry	Viral infections, childhood diseases, hives, herpes simplex, colds, flu, menstrual cycle, calms the nerves, nausea, and morning sickness.
Sarsaparilla	Boils, various infections, blood cleanser, and food poisoning.
Sassafras	Various infections, boils, blood cleanser, convulsions, and ear.
Saw Palmetto	Prostate problems.
Shepherd's Purse	Low backache and bleeding.
Skullcap	Nerves, chest, rabid bites, stings, and bites.
Spearmint	Nerves, convulsions, diarrhea, nausea, children's chills, and fever.
Spikenard	Backache and sluggishness.
Squaw Vine	Menstrual cramps.
St. John's Wort	Various bruises, injuries, damaged nerves, depression, pain, infections, menopause, and nervousness.

Tormentil Root	Hemorrhoids
Valerian Root	Nervous system, muscles, tension, convulsions, inflamed chest, stings, rabid animal and insect bites.
Vitamin A or D	Sand fly or flea bites, boils, pain, and bruises.
Vitamin E	Chiggers, other non-poisonous bites, circulation, lower back muscles, bruises, infections, and pain.
White Oak Bark	Gallstones, infections, bites, stings, snake bites, or bleeding.
White Willow Bark	External bleeding and pain.
Wild Yam	Colic, gas, indigestion, and pain.
Wintergreen Oil	Muscles and nervous system.
Wood Betony	Splinters.
Yarrow	Fevers from measles, colds, flu, or skin eruptions.

COMMERCIALLY PREPARED REMEDIES

REMEDY	PROBLEM
Adren-Aid	Anxiety, dizziness, exhaustion, flu, frostbite, hangover, motion sickness, or phobias.
AKN	Skincare Bedsores, boils, or insect repellent.
BF&C	Backache, various skin eruptions and abrasions, bones, chicken pox, fungus, gout, hemorrhoids, insect repellent, sciatic, teething, and teeth grinding.
BreatheAid	Allergies, asthma, coughing, fever, flu, or sinusitis.

Cal-Silica	Various skin abrasions and eruptions, diarrhea, eyes, gall bladder, gout, measles, cramps, nightmares, prostate, sciatica, teething, teeth, and ingrown toenail.
Ex-Stress	Anxiety, backache, intestinal problems, convulsions, depression, fainting, eyes, hiccups, nausea, insomnia, throat, shock, sprains, ulcers.
Fenu-Thyme	Asthma, colds, flu, congesting, fever, glandular swelling, throat, mumps, swollen glands, or sinusitis.
Kalmin	Various skin eruptions and abrasions, asthma, backache, convulsions, depression, fainting, diarrhea, fever, gall bladder, heart, hiccups, throat, chicken pox, insect repellent, insomnia, female organs and problems, nausea, vomiting, poisons, shock, nightmares, tonsils, ulcers, teething, and toothache.
Liquid Trace Minerals	For various skin eruptions and abrasions, rashes, blood poisoning, intestinal disorders, gall bladder, lice, burns, poisons, ears, eyes, childhood diseases, heart, bones, and teeth.
Liveron	Constipation, hangover, motion sickness, sty, tonsils, or warts.
Red Clover	Various bites and stings, fungus, hemorrhoids, Combination lice, prostate, stroke, testicles, or warts.
Rescue Remedy	Appendicitis, anxiety, rashes, abrasions and wounds, childhood diseases, eyes, hemorrhoids, hiccups, nausea, vomiting, shock, dizziness, cramps, convulsions, depression, burns, and toothache.

HERBAL SHOPPING LIST

This shopping sheet has been prepared to help you purchase the herbs you would like in your own natural remedy kit that fit the needs of your family. You can buy the herbs at your local health store. Single and combination herbs are only listed because they are easier to find, whereas homeopathics may not be as readily available, unless you have a homeopath in your immediate area. For commercially prepared homeopathic remedies, you can generally tell from the name what problems it helps.

The herbal remedy is listed on the left. You can check off on the right side which form is best suited to your needs. To administer your selected herbs, refer to the individual entry on the immediate problem for instructions.

HERB	CAPSULE	EXTRACT	TINCTURE	OINTMENT	OIL
Alfalfa	❑	❑	❑	❑	❑
Bayberry	❑	❑	❑	❑	❑
Black Walnut	❑	❑	❑	❑	❑
Burdock Root	❑	❑	❑	❑	❑
Catnip	❑	❑	❑	❑	❑
Chamomile	❑	❑	❑	❑	❑
Chickweed	❑	❑	❑	❑	❑
Cramp Bark	❑	❑	❑	❑	❑
Echinacea	❑	❑	❑	❑	❑
Eucalyptus Oil	❑	❑	❑	❑	❑
False or True Unicorn	❑	❑	❑	❑	❑

HERB	CAPSULE	EXTRACT	TINCTURE	OINTMENT	OIL
Fenugreek	❑	❑	❑	❑	❑
Feverfew	❑	❑	❑	❑	❑
Gravel Root	❑	❑	❑	❑	❑
Goldenseal	❑	❑	❑	❑	❑
Juniper Berry	❑	❑	❑	❑	❑
Lungwort	❑	❑	❑	❑	❑
Marigold	❑	❑	❑	❑	❑
Marshmallow	❑	❑	❑	❑	❑
Mistletoe	❑	❑	❑	❑	❑
Mullein	❑	❑	❑	❑	❑
Myrrh	❑	❑	❑	❑	❑
Pau D'arco	❑	❑	❑	❑	❑
Peppermint	❑	❑	❑	❑	❑
Red Clover	❑	❑	❑	❑	❑
Red Raspberry	❑	❑	❑	❑	❑
Sarsaparilla	❑	❑	❑	❑	❑
Skullcap	❑	❑	❑	❑	❑
Spearmint	❑	❑	❑	❑	❑
Squaw Vine	❑	❑	❑	❑	❑
St. John's Wort	❑	❑	❑	❑	❑
Valerian Root	❑	❑	❑	❑	❑

HERB	CAPSULE	EXTRACT	TINCTURE	OINTMENT	OIL
Vitamin A or D	❏	❏	❏	❏	❏
Vitamin E	❏	❏	❏	❏	❏
White Willow Bark	❏	❏	❏	❏	❏
Wild Yam	❏	❏	❏	❏	❏
Wintergreen Oil	❏	❏	❏	❏	❏
Adren-Aid	❏	❏	❏	❏	❏
AKN Skincare	❏	❏	❏	❏	❏
BF&C	❏	❏	❏	❏	❏
BreatheAid	❏	❏	❏	❏	❏
Cal-Silica	❏	❏	❏	❏	❏
Ex-Stress	❏	❏	❏	❏	❏
Fenu-Thyme	❏	❏	❏	❏	❏
Kalmin	❏	❏	❏	❏	❏
Liquid Trace Minerals	❏	❏	❏	❏	❏
Liveron	❏	❏	❏	❏	❏
Red Clover Combination	❏	❏	❏	❏	❏
Rescue Remedy	❏	❏	❏	❏	❏

OTHER _____

BOOKS TO READ

HERBAL REFERENCES

1. Bricklin, Mark. NATURAL HOME REMEDIES. PA: Rodale Press, 1982.
2. Christopher, John R. SCHOOL OF NATURAL HEALING. UT: BiWorld Publishers, 1976.
3. Christopher, John R. CHILDHOOD DISEASES. UT: Christopher Publishers, 1978.
4. Christopher, John R. EVERY WOMAN'S HERBAL. UT: Christopher Pub., 1987.
5. Jensen, Bernard. HERBAL HANDBOOK. CA: Jensen Publishers, 1988.
6. Kloss, Jethro. BACK TO EDEN. CA: Woodbridge Press, 1975.
7. Mabey, Richard. THE NEW AGE HERBALIST. NY: Macmillan Publishers, 1988.
8. Santillo, Humbart. NATURAL HEALING WITH HERBS. AZ: Hohm Press, 1985.
9. Shook, Edward. ELEMENTARY TREATISE IN HERBOLOGY. GA: Trinty Press, 1974.
10. Shook, Edward. ADVANCED TREATISE IN HERBOLOGY. GA: Trinty Press, 1978.
11. Stanway, Andrew. THE NATURAL FAMILY DOCTOR. NY: Simon & Schuster, 1987.
12. Tenney, Louise. TODAY'S HERBAL HEALTH. UT: Hawthorne Books, 1982.
13. Walker, N.W. RAW VEGETABLE JUICE. AZ: Norwalk Press, 1970.

HOMEOPATHIC REFERENCES

1. Cummings, Stephen and Ullman, Dana. EVERYBODY'S GUIDE TO HOMEOPATHIC MEDICINES. CA: Jeremy P. Tarcher, Inc, 1984.

2. Panos, Maesimund B. and Heimlich, Jane. HOMEOPATHIC MEDICINE AT HOME. CA: Jeremy P. Tarcher, Inc, 1980.

3. Vithoulkas, George. HOMEOPATHY: MEDICINE OF THE NEW MAN. NY: Arco Publishing, Inc, 1983.

REFERRALS
AND INFORMATION RESOURCES

American Association of Naturopathic Physicians (AANP)
2366 Eastlake Avenue
Suite 322
Seattle, WA 98102

(206) 323-7610

The AANP is a professional organization for naturopathic physicians. They can provide you with information on NDs in your area, what naturopathic medicine is and educational opportunities.

American Holistic Medical Association (AHMA)
4101 Lake Boone Trail
Suite 201
Raleigh, NC 27607

(919) 787-5146

The AHMA is a professional organization for medical doctors, naturopathic physicians, osteopathic physicians and chiropractors. All of their members practice or believe in the practice of natural medicine. They can give you the name of a physician who uses natural medicine in your area.

American Botanical Council (ABC)
PO Box 201660
Austin, TX 78720

(512) 331-8868

ABC is a group dedicated to the advancement of herbal or botanical medicine through education, research and political arenas. They publish a quarterly magazine called "HerbalGram" and sell booklets and books on herbalism.

The College of Maharishi Ayur-Veda Health Center
PO Box 282
Fairfield, IA 52556

(515) 472-5866

This center provides referrals to practitioners using Ayurvedic medicine. They also train practitioners and give out information to the public.

American Chiropractic Association (ACA)
1701 Clarendon Blvd
Arlington, VA 22209

(703) 276-8800

This group will refer you to a chiropractor in your area. They also publish a newsletter.

American Osteopathic Association (AOA)
142 East Ontario St
Chicago, ILL 60611

(312) 280-5800

The AOA can refer you to a DO in your town.

INDEX

A

Abdomen bandage, 38
Abdominal thrust, 72-73
Abscesses, 1-4
   peritonsillar, 233-35
Acidophilus, 250, 257
Activated charcoal, 93, 116
Agrimony, 209-10
Alcoholism, 133-34
   See also Hangover
Alfalfa, 39
Allergies, 5-8
   food, 5, 77
   See also Coughing; Eye problems
Allspice, 92
Almond nut milk, 102
Aloe vera, 2, 21-22, 25-26, 39, 41, 45,
   56, 58-59, 63, 68, 82, 105, 120,
   123, 166, 184, 198, 209, 217-18,
   220, 231-32, 244
Amenorrhea, 169
Ankle bandage, 35
Ankle splint, 53-55
Antifungal paste, 123
Anxiety, nervousness, or phobias, 8-11
Apoplexy, *See* Strokes
Appendicitis, 11-12
Apple, 109
Apple cider vinegar, 2, 14, 22, 26, 41,
   43, 45, 56, 63, 68, 75, 79, 87, 92,
   94-95, 98, 109, 112, 116, 131, 161,
   167, 178, 184, 198-99, 209, 212,
   215, 220, 223, 230, 232, 236, 244,
   248
Apple juice, 94-95, 128
Arterial bleeding, 29
Asthma, 12-15

Athlete's foot, 122, 123
Avocado oil, 199
Axillary temperature, 110

B

Backache, 17-20
Back bandage, 38
Bacteremia, *See* Blood poisoning
Baking soda, 26, 78-79, 115, 158, 176,
   184, 198, 242, 249
Bananas, 93
Bandaging techniques, 30-32
Barberry, 129
Barley, 112
Barley water, 93
Basil, 26, 183
Bayberry, 6, 59, 93, 221, 225, 234
Bedsores, 20-24
Beet juice, 171
Benign prostatic hyperplasia (BPH),
   192-93
Bent arm or elbow splint, 50-51
Biliary colic, 127
Bites and stings, 24-28
Black cohosh, 39, 171, 180
Black walnut, 23, 125, 167, 199, 234,
   237, 249
Black walnut extract, 3
Bleeding, 28-32
   ankle bandage, 35
   back, chest, abdomen, side ban-
     dages, 38
   bandaging techniques, 30-32
   chest bandage, 37
   direct pressure, 30-31
   finger and end of finger, bandage
     for, 32-33

ABOUT THE AUTHOR

James Kusick is a Naturopathic Consultant who has practiced for over 20 years with thousands of cases at his fingertips to refer to in compiling this book. He has a B.A. in Religion, a minor in Educational Psychology with a teacher's certificate from Stetson University, a Masters in Religious Education and Counseling from New Orleans Baptist Seminary, and a Doctorate of Ministry from Luther Rice Seminary. Under Dr. Christopher at the School of Natural Healing, Kusick earned his Master Herbalist and Iridology degrees, and taught there for 5 years. His degree in Advanced Iridology was awarded under the tutelage of Dr. Jensen in California. And Kusick has a doctorate in Counseling Psychology.

As a Naturopath, his specialty is Advanced Applied Kinesiology, Homeopathy, and special counseling and releasing techniques. In addition to his practice, he is currently on the Board of Directors of St. John's University in Springfield, LA and is an instructor in Religion, Metaphysics, and Parapsychology.

In his spare time for enjoyment, Kusick, a member of the Screen Actors Guild (SAG) and American Federation of Television and Radio Arts (AFTRA), enjoys acting in various plays, movies, and television commercials.